Instructor's Resource Manual

READING STRATEGIES FOR NURSING AND ALLIED HEALTH

D1546199

Instructor's Resource Manual

READING STRATEGIES FOR NURSING AND ALLIED HEALTH

Ann B. Faulkner
Brookhaven College

Dana K. Stahl
El Centro College

HOUGHTON MIFFLIN COMPANY   BOSTON   NEW YORK

Senior Sponsoring Editor: Mary Jo Southern
Senior Associate Editor: Ellen Darion
Editorial Assistant: Kate O'Sullivan
Manufacturing Manager: Florence Cadran
Senior Marketing Manager: Nancy Lyman

Contents

Preface

This Instructor's Manual for *Reading Strategies for Nursing and Allied Health* contains lesson plans, teaching tips, and unit tests that are based on the authors' classroom experience with this text over the last several years. We hope that the materials will make it easier for you to use this text with your students. We particularly hope that this manual will reduce any concern you may have felt about using nursing and allied health content to teach reading. Our experience shows that students like this process-centered approach to reading and that they really enjoy reading materials that relate to their future careers. It's more important for you to welcome students into a community of learners than it is to be an expert on this content.

The final part of each teaching tip contains the answers to quizzes and other activities that have "right answers." Although we are committed to the concept of a dialogue through the Consultation section, we agree with some of our reviewers that sharing the answers to tests in the textbook makes it too difficult for students to avoid the temptation to copy.

We certainly welcome your comments and those of your students about the "right answers" as well as the other suggestions we have included. We hope this manual contains sufficient clarifying information, and we look forward to any inquiries that can make you feel more comfortable with the various articles and text chapters.

Ann Faulkner
Brookhaven College

Dana K. Stahl
El Centro College

Instructor's Resource Manual

READING STRATEGIES FOR NURSING AND ALLIED HEALTH

Lesson Plan for a Fifteen-Week Semester

Week 1

- Introduce course, text, and vocabulary development.
- Introduce Unit 1, The Reading and Remembering Process. Focus on Before-Reading Strategies.
- Introduce Unit 2, Orientation to the Health Professions. Assign Selection 2-1, "Introduction to Physical Therapy."

Week 2

- Check Selection 2-1, "Introduction to Physical Therapy."
- Introduce and assign Selection 2-2, "The Birth of a New Profession."
- Introduce word parts and assign Latin roots.

Week 3

- Introduce Periodical Project and visit library's periodical collection.
- Check Selection 2-2, "The Birth of a New Profession," and introduce Selection 2-3, "Blessed Are the Flexible."
- Check Selection 2-3 and introduce Selection 2-4, "Chattering Hopes and Advices."

Week 4

- Check Selection 2-4 and introduce Selection 2-5, "Using an Index."
- Check Selection 2-5 and introduce Selection 2-6, "Cultural Considerations."
- Continue learning and reviewing Latin roots.

Week 5

- Check Selection 2-6.
- Review for test by sharing student-written multiple-choice questions on the publications.
- Review all Latin roots.
- Check progress on Periodical Project.
- *TEST 1:* Before-Reading Strategies, Unit 2: Orientation to the Health Professions, Latin roots, and personal vocabulary list.

Week 6

- Review Unit 1, The Reading and Remembering Process. Focus on During-Reading Strategies.
- Introduce Unit 3, Pain, and assign Selection 3-1, "Care of Patients with Pain."
- Return and discuss TEST 1.
- Introduce Greek roots.
- Continue work on Periodical Project.

Week 7

- Check Selection 3-1, "Care of Patients with Pain," and assign Selection 3-2, "Nurses Plunged Me Into the Pain Cycle; Nurses Pulled Me Out."
- Check Selection 3-2 and assign Selection 3-3, "Nurses' Judgments of Pain in Term and Preterm Newborns."
- Check Selection 3-3 and assign Selection 3-4, "Review of Literature on Culture and Pain of Adults, with Focus on Mexican-Americans."
- Turn in Periodical Project.
- Continue learning and reviewing Greek roots.

Week 8

- Check Selection 3-4 and assign Selection 3-5, "Avoiding Opioid-Induced Respiratory Depression."
- Check Selection 3-5.
- Review for test with students' multiple-choice questions, and review Greek roots.
- *TEST 2:* During-Reading Strategies, Unit 3: Pain, Greek roots, and personal vocabulary list.

Week 9

- Review Unit 1, The Reading and Remembering Process. Focus on After-Reading Strategies.
- Introduce Unit 4: Ethical and Legal Issues. Assign Selection 4-1, "Ethics and Values."
- Return and discuss TEST 2.
- Check Selection 4-1 and assign Before-Reading activities for Selection 4-2, "Ethical Perceptions of Parents and Nurses in NICU: The Case of Baby Michael."
- Introduce leisure-reading book report assignment and begin book selection process.

Week 10

- Introduce summaries, assign Selection 4-2, During- and After-Reading activities.
- Check Selection 4-2 and introduce outlining. Assign Selection 4-3, "Ethical Decision Making."
- Introduce Prefixes.
- Bring leisure-reading book to class. Begin reading.

Week 11

- Check Selection 4-3, introduce note-making, and assign Selection 4-4, "Caring for Pediatric Patients with HIV."
- Take quiz on Selection 4-4 in class.
- Continue learning and reviewing prefixes.
- Discuss book logs for one-quarter of book.
- Assign Selection 4-5, "When Language Is an Obstacle."

Week 12

- Check Selection 4-5.
- Review for test using students' multiple-choice questions.
- *TEST 3:* After-Reading Strategies, Unit 4: Ethical and Legal Issues, prefixes, and personal vocabulary list.
- Discuss book logs for one-half of book.

Week 13

- Review Unit 1, The Reading and Remembering Process. Focus on a review of all three phases.
- Introduce Unit 5: Stress. Assign Selection 5-1, "Stress."
- Check Selection 5-1, and assign Selection 5-2, "Stress and Anxiety."
- Discuss book logs for three-quarters of book.

Week 14

- Test covering Selection 5-2 in class. Assign Selection 5-3, "Analyzing Job Demands and Coping Techniques."
- Introduce Unit 6: Review and Practice in Critical Thinking. Choose assignments.
- Check Selection 5-3.
- Discuss book logs for the completed book. Review book report requirements.

Week 15

- Reports on Unit 6 assignments.
- Review for Final Exam.
- Share book reports informally.

Finals Week

- Final Exam
- Exit interviews

Teaching Tips

Unit 1: The Reading and Remembering Process

Unit 1 introduces the format of *Reading Strategies for Nursing and Allied Health (RSNAH)* and presents the Reading and Remembering Process that will be used through the remaining units. The strategies to be applied in each phase of the reading process are covered in activities that precede the "publication," which, in this unit, is the authors' essay on the Reading and Remembering Process.

Help students become familiar with the format for the text by pointing out where the article starts. Point out that the directions for what to do with the article are provided in the "Purpose for Reading" section as well as in the Before, During, and After Reading activities.

In the "Purpose for Reading" section there are two types of goal statements. The Process Goal refers to the reading process and focuses on one or more of the specific goals listed in the Reading and Remembering Process chart at the end of this first unit. The Outcome Goal indicates the results that students should expect to achieve as a result of studying the material. The Outcome Goal is similar to a classroom teacher's assignment for reading new material.

Although it is perfectly appropriate to look over all the activities before beginning the first one, students should be urged to do the activities in order. It may be tempting to skip to the "bottom line" and try to do the last activities without doing the earlier ones. This shortcut method undermines the application of a process for reading, which will ultimately enables students to get to "bottom lines" accurately and efficiently on many different assignments. The process should be mastered first.

Encourage students to check the Consultations section for a comparison of their answers to the two Before Reading questions before proceeding to the study planning activity. Before students make their first study plan, allow them to talk about the constraints on their study time *and* their responsibility to give studying a priority in their lives.

Although reading the essay on the Reading and Remembering Process may take place outside of class, encourage students to review their Outcome Goal before beginning. Encourage students to then push themselves to make notes and review the essay before considering themselves finished.

For this first assignment, ask students not to write their answers to the After Reading Quiz at home. Instead, encourage them to read over the questions, get their answers in mind, and then complete the quiz as a recall exercise during the next class. Following the quiz, ask students to compare their results with those in the Consultations section.

Following the Consultations check, students are probably ready for a discussion of the Reading and Remembering Process. Using a visual aid, such as a transparency of the chart or a computer-based presentation of the process, may help reinforce learning that occurred while reading and will aid recall of points needing clarification. The authors will be happy to provide a self-running presentation for Windows users for the cost of a disk and postage.

TESTING: No Unit Test has been prepared for this unit.

Unit 2: Orientation to the Health Professions

Phase 1: Before Reading

Unit 2 focuses on the goals and techniques of the Before Reading Process, but it includes activities for each of the three phases. By giving students extended practice with a variety of pre-reading strategies, the authors hope to impart a curiosity and involvement with the text that students often don't bring to studying. As the introduction to this unit points out, pre-reading techniques may be useful at times other than before reading. The recursive nature of the reading process may make it useful for a student to "get oriented" well after reading has begun—especially if the material presents unanticipated difficulties.

Because the publications included in this unit cover such a wide range of topics, special efforts may be necessary to keep students' concentration on the goals of learning how to get oriented to new material and learning how to plan for study. Consider reviewing the transparency or the computer-based presentation frequently. In subsequent units, the topics provide greater subject-matter coherence than they do here.

Selection 2-1: "Introduction to Physical Therapy"

Here, for the first time, students will have a chance to work on a textbook chapter from an allied health field: physical therapy. Much of the front matter of the text is included to allow students to simulate the initial exploration of a new textbook. Chapter 1 is typical of most health texts in providing an introduction to the profession in its opening pages. If your students have selected a different health major, they are encouraged to compare what they discover about physical therapy with what they know (or can look up) about their chosen field.

Again, helping students to see the demarcation between the activities and the pages from *Introduction to Physical Therapy* will be useful. Transparency Master 5 is included for the types of information to look for during the preview of a new textbook.

Students may need some help with the subtraction of time required for estimating elapsed time in reading. Here are a couple of examples that may be useful (see also Transparency Master 6):

	Stop time:	8:10 P.M.			Stop time:	9:00
minus	Start time:	7:00 P.M.		minus	Start time:	7:15
	Total time:	1:10 minutes			Total time:	1:45 (remember that 9:00 is the same as 8:60; don't try to borrow 100 minutes!)

Both of the During-Reading goals involve metacognition. This might be a good time to have a discussion of this self-analytical skill. Students sometimes deny that they are aware of checking on how they're doing while they're studying. Many realize that they have been getting internal feedback, but most of that feedback involves messages about inadequate performance and impending failure. Therefore, they don't want to hear such messages and may even stop studying to escape the bad news. When the internal analysis of performance is based on clear outcomes and is conducted frequently, metacognition is much more helpful. By becoming aware of whether they're getting what they need from reading, students give themselves a powerful tool to improve studying.

Stress the need to answer the three Review Questions from memory. Indeed, you might even ask students to write the three answers in class from memory to help them see how much information they are retaining.

TESTING: The Unit Test contains items relating to the identification of the author, the model definition's major sections, characteristics of a profession, and the part of a book useful for locating particular chapters. You may want to draw attention to these aspects of the chapter during class discussion without, of course, saying that these are the items to be tested.

Selection 2-2: "The Birth of a New Profession"

Most students will be reading a journal article for the first time. The article presents a history lesson on the development of radiologic technologists, so it does not contain highly technical vocabulary.

To help introduce the preview, you might hold up the book and page through the article while students look for the items to be included in the preview. Transparency Master 7 includes a list of items students should preview in an article. It is slightly more general than the list in the Before Reading activity. If time permits, students might answer the five Before Reading questions in class.

To build background knowledge, students are encouraged to use reference materials to learn something about x-rays, to orient themselves to events in 1895 (the year of the discovery of x-rays), and to come up with a milestone for each decade from the 1920s to the 1960s. Without any historical background, students will have much more difficulty integrating new information and remembering it. This is an ideal time to let students explore CD-ROM encyclopedias. *Encarta* has a timeline feature that will provide a clear picture of other things that were happening in 1895. *Time Almanac of the 20th Century* covers the 1920s through the present with articles, videos, pictures, and maps.

TESTING: Test questions over this article include identifying the authors' background, the role of Elizabeth Ascheim, the effect of both world wars on the profession, and the date on which the authors indicate that the term *radiologic technologist* had become accepted.

"Right Answers"
After Reading 2

GOAL: *Periodically test recall of relevant information*
TECHNIQUE: *Answer possible test questions*

1. The need for a special uniform to distinguish x-ray personnel from other hospital workers was suggested in the *1930s.*

2. In the *1950s,* the need for training in testing equipment and making minor repairs became apparent.

3. Among the first x-ray operators was *Elizabeth Ascheim,* who made many contributions to the development of the profession although she died at age *(from 1859 to 1905 is) 46 years* because she failed to take the necessary precautions to prevent her own exposure. (Taking time to do this subtraction when you read is a good idea; it makes the point about her untimely death very clear. But you might be excused for misspelling her name!)

4. By the 1940s, the job duties of the ideal professional were recognized as so complex and demanding as to suggest that anyone who fulfilled them deserved *wings.* (Any answer suggesting angel-status gets the idea conveyed on page 41.)

5. The group now known as the American Society of Radiologic Technologists was founded in the *1920s,* with the assistance of Ed Jerman. (This answer took close reading of the introductory sentence in the "Early Technician Training" section on page 42.)

6. By the *1960s,* radiological professionals were required to receive training that provided both technical expertise and ethical understanding.

7. During the 1920s, various people in physicians' offices performed the job that came to be known as x-ray *technician.*

Selection 2-3: "Blessed Are the Flexible . . ."

It might be useful to check this book out from your library to introduce it to the class. The role of a book's foreword is easier to understand when it's seen in context, and looking at the table of contents (which is not included in our text) will show where this particular essay appears.

Remind students that the focus of all activities in Unit 2 is to explore pre-reading techniques. This publication represents another type of writing: collected writings of a prominent author.

This article also gives students an insight into the history of a health field: nursing. The purpose here is pleasure rather than academic reading. Instead of reading to remember benchmark events in each decade, students are encouraged to have a good time while learning about the author's style.

If it hasn't already come up, you'll probably have to discuss how close students need to come to the response in the Consultations in order to consider themselves to have the "right answer." Ask several students to share their statements of the main idea from the second Before Reading Activity, and help them analyze the characteristics of an accurately stated main idea. Remind them that at the Before Reading stage, mental involvement with the text is more important than word-for-word accuracy.

Students will have a good time talking about the new and amusing points in the article, especially the 1905 list. Encourage the students to relate this information to what they know about radiologic technology at the same period of time.

TESTING: The Unit Test includes items on the introduction of the article's author by the foreword's author, on the suggestions that Curtin makes for nurses, and on the 1905 list of "Rules for Nurses."

Selection 2-4: "Chattering Hopes and Advices"

Florence Nightingale will challenge your students. Taking a little time to build an appreciation for her role in history is worthwhile. The facsimile edition of her 1859 publication is probably available in your library, and students will understand more about its original format and style if they can see it. Again, encyclopedias, especially on CD-ROM, will be useful in helping students develop background for understanding the context in which Nightingale wrote.

Students may have trouble "seeing" the outline of the article presented in the third Before Reading activity. You might do the filling in and paraphrasing in class to help students understand what can be gained from thinking about the author's main ideas before reading.

Warn students not to skip footnotes, and help them see where the notes are and how each one relates to the text.

Encourage students to use their best writing process on the final After-Reading activity. Prewriting, drafting, and revising closely parallel the three phases of the reading process. Alert students to your expectation that this essay will reflect their best work on each phase of their writing.

TESTING: There are four questions on the Unit Test from this publication. One asks students to recognize the paraphrase of a heading (emphasizing the avoidance of three words in a row from the original). Others involve background about the times in which Nightingale wrote, her suggestions for pleasing the sick, and some of her advice that seems wrong, given our current understanding of contagion.

After Reading 3

GOAL: *Organize relevant information for review*
TECHNIQUES: *Think critically about what you have learned*

Your response may reflect a very different reaction to Nightingale's ideas, but it should follow this general form: (1) Indicate your general reaction to the ideas in the chapter (positive or negative); (2) list specific examples of Nightingale's dos and don'ts that determine your general reaction; and (3) indicate any contrasting reactions you have to particular parts of Nightingale's chapter.

1. For one-hundred-forty-year-old advice, Florence Nightingale's suggestions to visitors of the sick are surprisingly fresh and useful.

2a. She seems to have the best interest of patients at heart when she advises against giving falsely cheerful, thoroughly impractical suggestions for getting well.
2b. She is also convincing in arguing against unrealistic wishes for a speedy recovery or long life to a terminally ill patient.
2c. The suggestions on ways to please the sick, especially the chronically ill, are excellent: share good news, don't cry or preach, let them have and care for a pet or have babies visit.

3. On the other hand, Nightingale seems to have no awareness of infectious disease processes. Babies don't need to be around TB patients, and energetic puppies would not be helpful to post-surgical patients.

Selection 2-5: "Using an Index"

The focus is on finding relevant material from the index of a textbook, and it may take some explaining to help students understand the task; nursing faculty report that many students have difficulty with using an index. Presenting students with textbooks from several allied health courses will help. Allied health faculty serving on textbook selection committees are good candidates for lending examination copies of their texts. Plan to transport them in several trips; many of the books are huge, especially in nursing.

Ask the students to work in pairs to find relevant information on pain, ethics, and stress. Once they are familiar with using the index, they will find it easier to use the five index sources reprinted here to locate information on patient teaching.

Although patient teaching is a common topic in nursing programs, the phrase *patient teaching* is not contained in either of the indexes. Students will be asked to think of synonyms for each key term in order to explore all the possibilities each text offers. Again, providing some in-class practice on synonyms is useful: Ask students to brainstorm other key words to use for searches on *pain*. For example, *comfort* is an antonym, but it is often used in nursing to introduce a discussion on how to avoid pain.

TESTING: There is only one question on the Unit Test that relates to the use of indexes. It asks students to pick synonyms for a phrase that might be the subject of an index search.

Selection 2-6: "Cultural Considerations"

Two articles from a student nursing association's magazine will present a moderate challenge while providing new information to discuss. Students will use previewing as a technique for deciding which of the two articles to read first. The outcome goal is to look for similarities and differences between the two client populations: African-Americans and Asian-Americans.

You may want to make and share notes on the two articles to let your students see that studying is not a matter of photographic memory—even "experts" need to make notes in order to remember complicated material.

If the class is fortunate enough to have some ethnic diversity, students may be able to validate, qualify, and extend the ideas presented by the two authors.

TESTING: There are four questions on the Unit Test relating to this pair of articles. From the Douglas article, students are asked to recognize a definition of cultural competence and to list efforts to close disparities in health outcomes. From the Louie article, students answer questions about the health risks of AAPIs and about nursing interventions appropriate to that group.

"Right Answers"
After Reading 4

GOAL: Test recall of relevant information
TECHNIQUE: Answer possible test questions

1. What is a "culturally competent nurse," according to Douglas? Do you think Louie would agree with that definition? Why?

   According to Douglas, a "culturally competent nurse" is aware and appreciative of cultural differences and how they affect the nursing process. Such a nurse tries to understand the cultural context of behavior. Louie would probably agree with this definition. She concludes with advice to understand the client's perspective on health issues and to incorporate traditional practices into the health care process.

2. Douglas includes three examples of cross-cultural differences that might produce misunderstandings between African-American clients and majority-culture health care providers. Explain each one.

The use of first names is used by majority-culture caregivers to establish rapport, but the African-American client may respond with humiliation to this sign of disrespect. Making eye contact with the listener is uncomfortable for some African-Americans although majority-culture caregivers may view the lack of eye contact as a sign of subservience or fear. Limiting hospital visitations to "immediate family only" may cause problems for African-Americans. They often view "instrumental" and "emotional support-givers" from their extended family as essential visitors. Majority-culture caregivers may view such people as "outsiders."

3. One culturally-related risk factor clearly affects the health of many African-Americans. Explain.

   The fatty diet of Southerners (where a majority of African-Americans lived until World War II) is a clear risk factor for diseases that may not show up until old age.

4. List four significant health issues for the African-American population, and indicate the health care response proposed by Douglas.

   Douglas says that the infant mortality rate (which is currently twice as high as that of the majority culture) could be reduced by prenatal care. Condom use in every sexual encounter would reduce the growing rate of AIDS among heterosexual African-American women exposed to AIDS by IV drug users and others. Substance abuse might be counteracted by offering health education to clergy. Hypertension might be reduced if church members were trained to take blood pressure readings and make appropriate referrals.

5. List four significant health issues for Asian-Americans and Pacific Islanders as a group. Where possible, indicate the health care response proposed by Louie.

   Louie points out problems in collecting and generalizing about information from this diverse group, but several issues do emerge as problems: cancer, hepatitis B, tuberculosis, and mental health problems, among others. Although no specific suggestions are made for lowering risk to the many types of cancer, educational programs covering diet and smoking would be helpful. Screening and treatment for hepatitis and TB, especially if community based, would be helpful. Louie's suggestions for responding to the mental health issues include adaptation of traditional attitudes and care in the use of culturally inappropriate norm groups. (You may well have chosen other items from Louie's list of nine, but suggestions for interventions are made from the items included at the end of the article.)

6. List six different subgroups within the AAPI group, and indicate a distinguishing health problem for each subgroup.

   (1) The South East Asian Refugees (Vietnamese, Laotians, and Cambodians) often approach illness as an imbalance of forces (yin/yang or hot/cold). They also use traditional remedies such as rubbing with a coin to induce fever.

   (2) The Vietnamese have a high incidence of dental and eye problems, along with high blood pressure.

   (3) The Chinese (who make up 24 percent of the AAPI group) must be differentiated by several factors including place of birth, dialect, and degree of acculturation. For many TB, hepatitis B, and cancer are health problems.

(4)   The indigenous Hawai'ians (Kanaka Maoli) are threatened with extinction in less than 50 years because of health and economic problems.

(5)   Asian Indians have very high rates of coronary artery disease because of their diet, smoking, and possibly some genetic factors.

(6)   Koreans include children adopted by U.S. families and bicultural families. They combine Western and traditional methods to address problems such as cancer, hepatitis B, and TB.

7.   What are some similarities in nursing interventions to provide culturally appropriate care, as suggested by Douglas and Louie?

> Both authors suggest that access is an issue: Louie directly suggests that neighborhood health care is needed for AAPI communities. Douglas proposes an institutional approach to access through the church. Louie's suggestions for the types of care needed include maternal/child care that is similar to Douglas's call for prenatal care for African-American women.

8.   What are some differences in the two authors' approaches to nursing interventions for the two groups? What's your explanation for the differences?

> Largely because the specific health care issues are different, the two authors' suggested interventions are different. Louie does not mention AIDS or substance abuse (except for smoking, which does not appear on Douglas's list) as major problems among the AAPI population. Douglas does not propose solutions for TB or hepatitis B problems because they are apparently not major risks to the African-American population.

9.   Does socioeconomic status affect the health status of African-Americans and Asian-American/Pacific Islanders equally, according to the two authors?

> Douglas makes clear the effect of poverty in individuals regardless of race (the death rate is three to seven times higher). She points out that African-Americans are often the most acculturated of the diverse cultures. Nevertheless, according to Douglas, "race is often used as a marker for poverty in terms of health outcomes." Louie, on the other hand, quotes a source showing that socioeconomic status is less important than lifestyle and cultural factors in explaining health differences among groups.

10.   Do you have any questions, based on your reading of the two articles? What are they?

> Do the differences in approach to the poverty versus culture debate mentioned in Question 9 form a real difference between the two authors? Can anyone make suggestions about how to avoid cancer (other than stopping smoking and reducing fat intake)?

Unit 3: Pain

Phase 2: During Reading

The process goals in Unit 3 introduce and provide practice in comprehension strategies and in monitoring reading efficiency. The publications focus on the subject of pain, and they tend to have a mutually reinforcing effect. As a result, students really develop expertise on the topic. Perhaps for the first time in their schooling, they become "academic insiders" when they recognize topics and authors from previous readings they have done in the unit. Then, too, almost everyone has had some contact with pain, either personally or through a close family member or friend. Students may hold some nonscientific attitudes toward pain, but they have fewer deficits in background knowledge on this topic than on the others in *RSNAH*.

Selection 3-1: "Care of Patients with Pain"

Just as they did with the chapter on physical therapy, the students will use the textbook-provided materials to guide and check their understanding of main ideas. Marking main ideas and noting organizational patterns are the process goals for the selection.

If you have time, do the Before Reading activities in class. They don't take much time, and they tend to be completed more thoroughly when done in a group.

You may want to demonstrate the underlining technique described in the first During Reading activity. Help students to focus on underlining only one main idea sentence per paragraph, leaving details for a later time.

You'll probably have material from another textbook that presents sample paragraphs for the various types of paragraph organization. It may be more helpful to use examples from the articles already covered in this text. For example, students used *comparison/contrast* in thinking about physical therapy as a profession. Florence Nightingale indicates a number of *effects* on patients of inappropriate conversation by their visitors; she also suggests several *causes* of improved morale for the sick. The article on the history of radiologic technologists uses *chronological order*. The 1905 *list* of rules for nurses will probably be recalled by most students. The list of organizational patterns is available as Transparency Master 8.

Accuracy rather than speed should be the paramount concern for most of our students. The goal of monitoring reading efficiency should not be viewed as an invitation to "speed reading." On the other hand, some of our ADHD (Attention Deficit/Hyperactivity Disorder) students have really improved their concentration by setting goals that are *slightly* faster than their current rate and by reading to meet those goals.

Although you may not have time to do an in-class test of retention, you might want to follow up the final After Reading activity with a quick check. Have the students number themselves from one to eight, then ask each student to answer the objective corresponding to their number. Transparency Master 9 provides a list of the eight objectives.

14

TESTING: In the Unit Test, students are asked to choose a definition of pain, to recall a detail about chronic pain, to recognize a fact about Melzack's Gate Control Theory, to recall the factors used in assessment of pain, and to select appropriate interventions for certain patients.

"Right Answers"
After Reading 3

GOAL: *Check initial recall of relevant information*
TECHNIQUE: *Review the whole assignment by self-testing*

The answers to the objective are expressed in terms of their location in the Study Outline on pages 107–110. Your wording will be unique, of course.

1. Define pain.

    I.A., B.

2. Describe physiologic and psychological reactions to pain stimuli.

    Physiologic: I.D.1, 4.
    Psychologic: I.D.5.

3. Compare and contrast three different types of pain.

    Table 10-1 Acute and Chronic Pain, p. 101.
    Figure 10-1 Referred pain, anterior and posterior views, p. 99.
    (Did you list something different? Referred pain seemed like the best choice for the third type of pain, but it is not clearly indicated in the text.)

4. Describe common biases and myths about pain.

    III.A.1–4.

5. Assess pain in assigned patients, fully appreciating the subjective nature of pain.

    Subjective data: III.B.1–5.
    Objective data: III.C.1.a, b and 2.

6. List at least seven nursing interventions other than the administration of analgesics for the relief of pain.

    If you use Table 10-2, include seven items between "cold packs and TENS units." The outline includes a 6-item list at IV.C.5.d. If you use the section Managing Other Chronic Pain, the outline lists 10 nonchemical methods at IV.C.6.a.

7. Select nursing interventions appropriate for each type of pain experience.

    Your answer here will depend on what you selected as "each type of pain experience." If you used the chronic/acute approach, your answer will come from Table 10-2, p. 104. If you thought of cancer pain and other chronic pain, your answer will come from IV.C.5 and 6 in the outline.

8. Evaluate the effectiveness of measures used for the management of pain in assigned patients.

(1) Anne Mays has chronic neck pain for which a muscle relaxant is prescribed. A muscle relaxant is designed to relax muscles, which will tend to reduce pain, but it is not a narcotic or an analgesic. Thus, the patient's fears of addiction are misplaced; she needs to be told about the purpose of her medication and its lack of addictive properties. Ms. Mays's pain might also be lessened through relaxation, massage, or biofeedback. Imagery might also be helpful. The possibility of using a TENS unit should be explored. To learn more about these techniques, I'd investigate special training in pain management.

(2) I'd ask the nurse going off duty if she's seen signs that Mr. Davis's pain is unsatisfactorily managed under current orders. If not, I'd pursue the placebo issue no further because the possibilities for cynical second-guessing about a patient's pain seem great with placebo therapy. Mr. Abernathy seems to be a placebo-positive responder, but there's no evidence that Mr. Davis would have the same response to saline. On the other hand, affirming the benefit of back rubs, massage, and the application of heat and cold while administering such treatments may enhance their benefit. All sorts of pleasurable experience facilitate endorphin relief, so music therapy, humor, or distraction may all produce a pain-lowering effect.

Selection 3-2: "Nurses Plunged Me Into the Pain Cycle; Nurses Pulled Me Out"

Students generally find this article interesting and easy to read. It's fun to contrast the treatment in the two facilities.

The first After Reading activity may need special explanation because of the inclusion of factors from the previous reading. Help students understand how they use the factors to label the contrasts between the two health care facilities.

The differences between the specialized definition of sympathy and the nontechnical definition are surprising. For health care providers, sympathy involves an inappropriate involvement of feelings coupled with inactivity; for the rest of us, sympathy provides a feeling of harmony with another, which may lead to greater understanding.

TESTING: The four test questions include identification of the author, the author's purpose, an application of the technical definition of pain, and the author's conclusion.

"Right Answers"
After Reading 4

GOAL: Organize relevant information for review
TECHNIQUE: Look up and learn new terms discovered during reading

1. j	6. f	10. b
2. d	7. c	11. k
3. g	8. i	12. m
4. e	9. h	13. l
5. a		

Selection 3-3: "Nurses' Judgments of Pain in Term and Preterm Newborns"

This is the first research article that most students have seen. Many of the terms used in research design will be unfamiliar. Transparency Master 10 shows a chart comparing the editor's outline with the author's is included to allow for some discussion of the meaning of terms. Transparency Master 10 will also facilitate the assignment to draw lines to connect the related terms.

Statistical analysis paralyzes some students. Try to help them see that the statistical conclusions are expressed in words; they don't have to become mathematicians to understand the author's ideas. In addition, the point of reading this article is to understand main ideas not statistics.

Transparency Master 11 is included to show the three reading strategies: skimming, selective reading, and comprehension reading.

Indicate to students that they are not actually required to prepare or deliver an oral report. (For many, reassurance on this score can save some sleeplessness.) On the other hand, asking students to share introductory or concluding observations that they identified in the final After Reading activity is not very threatening and often proves quite interesting.

TESTING: The three test questions include identification of the author's objective, recognizing a statement of the results of the study, and selecting the best summary of the selection.

"Right Answers"
After Reading 1

GOAL: Check initial recall of relevant information
TECHNIQUE: Review the whole assignment by self-testing

Objective/Purpose

Carla Shapiro's *purpose* was to examine nurses' assessment of pain in preterm and full-term newborns. She also wanted to discover what clues the nurses used to determine whether the infants in each group were experiencing pain.

Design/Methods

Working with Canadian nurses in a neonatal intensive care unit, Shapiro's *methods* included showing videotapes of babies getting a heel lance and asking the nurses to rate the pain on a line from no pain to the most intense pain possible. She also asked the nurses to list the clues used to assess the baby's pain.

Conclusions/Implications, Limitations, Recommendations, Results

Her *results* showed that the nurses thought the full-term babies were experiencing more pain than the preemies. There were less significant differences in the pain clues for the two groups of babies. From these results, she *concluded* that the "vigor and richness" of a baby's pain response affects how much pain the nurse thinks the baby has. Shapiro *recommends* additional education for nurses on these topics.

Selection 3-4: "Review of Literature on Culture and Pain of Adults, with Focus on Mexican-Americans"

This article does not present original research; rather, it summarizes and evaluates the research of others. It may be helpful to know that for one of our students, the article proved the key to understanding a very bewildering experience she had as an aide in a dentist's office. The Anglo dentist had often seemed upset and irritated by the groans of his Hispanic, especially female Hispanic, patients. He seemed to feel that the patients' groans were signaling a need for greater pain medication or at least a wish that he would stop hurting them. If patients denied that they wanted more pain killer or indicated that he should continue with the procedure, the dentist became angry and sometimes refused to continue work with a groaning patient. The student, an aide who was also an Hispanic female, tried to suggest that she didn't think the groaning was a complaint or a request. She felt that it merely allowed the patient to vent. Although she had been unsuccessful in her transcultural communication efforts with the dentist, she felt profoundly vindicated by the research in this article. In fact, she commented that this was the first time she had read anything by an author who had clearly been in "her neighborhood."

Help students sort out stereotypes from research-based generalizations. Without careful reading, students who harbor stereotypes about Hispanics' responses to pain will miss qualifiers in the text or even completely misread the authors' findings. Your best opportunity to do this will be in discussing the main ideas students listed for each section of the article.

The invitation to look for familiar names in the bibliography is designed to give students a chance to realize that they are no longer beginners in reading pain literature. McCaffery, whose definition of pain opened the text chapter, is writing here with a co-author, Meinhart, but her name is worth recognizing. It will appear again!

TESTING: There are four test questions on this article. One asks students to identify the type of article; two ask about details from the literature review, and one asks about implications.

"Right Answers"
After Reading 1

GOAL: Check initial recall of relevant information
TECHNIQUE: Review the whole assignment by self-testing

To check your work, re-read the abstract at the beginning of the article and the sentences you underlined in the "Implications" and "Recommendations" sections. Are your translations of the authors' underlinings similar to these?

Implications

Nurses need to know about culture and pain in general and specifically about traditional beliefs and practices.

Assessing a patient's pain must consider adherence to traditional beliefs, as well as the meaning and function of pain-related behaviors such as crying and moaning.

The type of intervention the patient wants should also be taken into consideration.

Recommendations

Problems with research methods make it important to conduct future research carefully.

More research is needed that qualitatively describes Mexican- and Anglo-American culture related to pain and quantitatively compares the two groups in various ways.

Cross-cultural assessment tools are also needed.

Selection 3-5: "Avoiding Opioid-Induced Respiratory Depression"

Although this article includes a test for continuing education credit, it is not beyond the comprehension of our students. Indeed, the biggest challenge is learning to pronounce *opioid* without stammering. But the successful mastery of the article and its test items will give students a real measure of their improvement.

One hint that might help students answer the questions in the first After Reading activity as well as in the author's test is *don't skip the boxes.* Valuable information is contained in the graphics and text boxes, particularly in the "Nine Ways to Prevent . . ." sidebar.

TESTING: The Unit Test includes questions on the definition of respiratory depression, on risk factors, and on monitoring and classifying the sedation level.

"Right Answers"
After Reading 1

GOAL: Organize relevant material for review
TECHNIQUE: Look up and learn new terms discovered during reading

1. What (exactly) do these abbreviations stand for?

   COPD
   chronic obstructive pulmonary disease (for example, emphysema)

   NSAID
   nonsteroidal anti-inflammatory drugs (defined on p. 152 in the box). If you can't provide examples of NSAIDs, you don't have enough information yet.

   PACU
   postanesthesia care unit

   PCA
   patient-controlled analgesia

   PRN
   pro re nata, in Latin; as needed, in English

   Where can you look up such abbreviations?

   Although PCA was introduced in Chapter 10 at the beginning of this unit, and COPD is in a recent college dictionary, such abbreviations will only be explained in a medical dictionary.

2. Use the chart on opioid characteristics on page 151 to answer these questions:

   a. Which opioid has the quickest onset time using the intravenous route?
   Fentanyl seems to be the fastest with any route, but the IV route is faster than epidural.

b.   Which opioid takes the longest time to reach peak of efficiency? Using which route?
Although it has a slow onset, the longest peak by far is obtained with morphine through an oral route.

c.   If the goal is delayed onset of analgesia, which medication and route would you recommend?
The slowest onset could be achieved by using oral morphine, but epidural morphine is almost as slow.

3.   If the "incidence of clinically significant respiratory depression in hospitalized adults receiving opioids in therapeutic doses is approximately 0.09%," how many people are affected?

$$0.09\% = .0009 = 9 \text{ of } 10,000 = \text{Answer c}$$

4.   Identify two factors that increase the risk for opioid-induced respiratory depression.

The risk of respiratory depression is greater for patients who are opioid naive (they have not taken opioids for a week or more) and for those who are opioid sensitive, which is hard to identify except through previous history.

"Right Answers After Reading 2

GOAL: *Test recall of relevant information*
TECHNIQUE: *Answer test questions*

The following list of "answers" is offered only as a basis for comparison and discussion among classmates. You are not eligible for the continuing education units offered by *AJN*, and these answers are not to be considered official or necessarily correct.

1.	a	6.	a	10.	c
2.	d	7.	a	11.	a
3.	b	8.	d	12.	c
4.	a	9.	a	13.	b
5.	c				

If you have a different answer, can you support it with a clear reference from the article? If so, can you convince others of your position? Can you give evidence showing that other answer choices are incorrect?

Unit 4: Ethical and Legal Issues

Phase 3: After Reading

Those in the health care field will interact daily with life or death issues. Thus, ethical and legal issues become a crucial topic in training students to work in this field. In Unit 4, the publications interrelate in such a way that students begin to develop a feeling of expertise, or at least familiarity, with legal and ethical issues.

The process goals in this unit stress After Reading activities. For many students, the idea of doing anything beyond highlighting while reading is new. Separating note-making from reading may seem inefficient if the goal is merely to get to the end of the chapter, but when students focus on the need to review material for a unit test and for comprehensive finals, note-making becomes a more relevant skill. The After Reading activities also include practice in outlining, paraphrasing, and summarizing. All three skills have their place as aids to recall, although they may also be taught as writing skills.

Selection 4-1: "Ethics and Values"

The introductory textbook chapter presents a variety of new terms, but memorizing them is not required. Instead, students are challenged to make very good in-text notes in order to pass an open-book test with at least 80 percent accuracy. To ensure students a chance to test their notes, you might paperclip the test pages together so that students won't see the actual test before they get to class. Obviously, they could remove the clip, but usually students will respond honorably to the challenge not to peek until it's time.

TESTING: There is a question on the definition of ethics and one on the definition of a moral dilemma. Students are asked to recall moral principles and to make an application of deontology.

"Right Answers"
After Reading 3

GOAL: *Test recall of relevant information*
TECHNIQUE: *Answer test questions*

Open Book Test Answers

1.	g	6.	h
2.	i	7.	c
3.	j	8.	b
4.	a	9.	f
5.	d	10.	k

Were your essay answers something like these? Certainly your examples will be different, but do they illustrate the same concept?

11. Utilitarianism is a Teleological Theory that focuses on consequences. It asks what action will provide "the greatest good or happiness for the greatest number." This doesn't mean that everyone will be happy but that the greatest number will be benefited. An example of a situation to illustrate utilitarianism is a decision that a particular drug should be put on the market for use to treat a disabling condition, even though 1 in 5,000 users experiences severe side effects. The use of the drug will make 4,999 people "happy" and only one will be "unhappy." Therefore, the consequences of the use of the drug will benefit the greatest number so the "right thing" is to release the drug for use.

12. The deontological theory focuses on rules or principles that guide action. The person who applies this theory says that decisions should be based on these principles. An example might be the person who says that all decisions should be based on the Golden Rule, "do unto others as you would have others do unto you." In contrast, utilitarian theory says that the decision should be based only on what the outcome will be—what will make the most people happy. In other words, what will benefit the greatest number of people. One person is guided by rules they live by, the other by rational decision regarding the best outcome. The result is that each person may come to different conclusions in a given situation. Nurses need to be able to deal with clients who make decisions based on ethical principles that are different from their own. Health professionals need to recognize that such decisions are valid for the particular client and therefore deserve to be honored.

13. Code 1: The nurse provides services with respect for human dignity and the uniqueness of the client—unrestricted by considerations of social or economic status, personal attributes, or the nature of the health problems.

   An example of this code occurs when a nurse is assigned to care for a man accused of murder. The patient is handcuffed to the bed with a guard at the bedside. The nurse might be horrified at the murder, but he/she must not let that affect the care given to the accused patient. The care the nurse gives him should be just as careful, just as good, and of the same quality of care given to any other patient in the hospital. In other words, the nurse can't alter nursing care because he/she doesn't like something about a patient.

14. Code 2: The nurse safeguards the client's right to privacy by judiciously protecting information of a confidential nature.

   The nurse must protect the patient's right to privacy by not giving out information about them or their care to anyone not involved in their care. The nurse can't discuss the specific patient with family or friends. The nurse must also make sure that anything said to another nurse about the patient will not be overheard by any person other than those involved in giving patient care.

15. Code 3: The nurse acts to safeguard the client and the public when health care and safety are affected by the incompetent, unethical, or illegal practice of any person.

If a nurse observes another nurse not taking care to protect a patient, the nurse must intervene in an appropriate way to prevent the injury. If a nurse notices that a nurse is drunk, the drunk nurse must be removed from patient care so no patient will be injured by the altered thinking and actions of the affected nurse.

16. Code 5: The nurse maintains competence in nursing.

Nurses must keep up-to-date with new medicines, treatments, and procedures; and they must continue to attend educational meetings, read journals, and so on to make sure their knowledge, skills, and care are current and safe.

17. Code 11: The nurse collaborates with members of the health professions and other citizens in promoting community and national efforts to meet the health needs of the public.

Nurses should participate in community service organizations to address the health of the public. They might volunteer in screening clinics, give talks about health issues in community centers, or volunteer in community health fairs. They may also participate in the dialog about current health care issues.

How did you do? Were the notes you made helpful in locating the information needed on the test? Think about how you can do better note-making next time.

Students who miss more than three answers have not performed at the required 80 percent level.

Selection 4-2: "Ethical Perceptions of Parents and Nurses in NICU: The Case of Baby Michael"

The critical activity for this publication is the last one. It requires a comprehensive summary of the article. Although it may be getting late in the semester, don't let students avoid doing a good job with this assignment. They will learn a great deal about their own comprehension by observing which aspects of the article were easy or hard to summarize. The most useful hint to give students as an aid to summarizing is to look at the graphics. In Tables 1 and 2 the authors provide a summary of their own work, which, if not ignored, can make students' summaries much easier to write.

TESTING: On the Unit Test, students are asked to recall the overall structure of the main ideas in the article, to provide an example of caring strategies, to recognize the details of Baby Michael's history, and to choose the best paraphrase of a key sentence, again avoiding the repetition of three words in a row from the original while remaining faithful to the meaning of the original.

"Right Answers"
After Reading 4

GOAL: Organize relevant information for review
TECHNIQUE: Summarize

Does your summary contain some of the following information?

Miya and her coauthors present the case of Baby Michael, a premature infant who might have permanent or overwhelming injury when he experienced complications of *intracranial* bleeding, cardiac arrest, *pneumothorax,* and *sepsis* on top of his already small size and immaturity. The parents and the nurses experienced many ethical challenges around the issues of treatment versus nontreatment, informed consent, and decision making. For example, the parents were generally overwhelmed by the NICU and believed nurses who suggested that Michael's only problem was that he "needed to grow." They felt sure that all the treatment Michael received in the NICU was routine and appropriate in their son's case. On the other hand, the nurses had the background to anticipate months of hospitalization and possible disabilities for Michael. Furthermore, they often felt that the treatment decisions led to more pain for the baby.

The suggestions for nursing interventions bring together techniques for crisis intervention with a 5-step caring process designed to help nurses realize their obligation to facilitate parents' right to informed decision making about their children. Suggestions include helping parents to express their feelings, to understand more about the situation, and to learn how to cope. The caring process involves knowing, being emotionally present, doing for, enabling, and maintaining belief in one's ability to get through the crisis.

Note: The italicized words are technical terms used in the article. Were you able to use some of them in your summary? It is a good idea to incorporate new technical terms in your writing—if you can use them correctly.

Selection 4-3: "Ethical Decision Making"

The selection of a chapter from this reference book was mandated by the discovery of the condition of our library's copy. Students had nearly thumbed this volume to pieces, indicating the usefulness of the resource in preparing for their classes.

Students will use information about Baby Michael in the previous publication to complete a chart like one in the text. They will also make an outline. Students are encouraged not to be overly concerned with traditional outline format but to use indentations to show the relative importance of ideas. Sharing your own outline may be very instructive for students. It will also be helpful to let them know if there were spots where you were unsure about whether to include a topic or how to paraphrase the author's words.

TESTING: Students answer four questions pertaining to this chapter. They involve comprehension of ambiguous issues, application of decision categories, application of a definition to a situation, and recognizing the consequences of an ethical position.

"Right Answers"
After Reading 2

GOAL: Organize relevant information for review
TECHNIQUES: Think critically about what you have learned; apply principles to real-life situations

Compare your choices with these and the ones listed in your chapter. Are they similar? Do you understand the difference? If not, you may want to reread sections of the chapter and discuss this with other students or with your instructor.

Type 1	**Type 2**
Nursing actions are both ethical and legal.	Nursing actions *may be considered* ethical but not legal.
Teaching Baby Michael's parents how to care for him after he leaves the hospital.	Increasing Baby Michael's medication to provide him with additional pain relief without a doctor's order.
Type 3	**Type 4**
Nursing actions *may be considered* legal but not ethical.	Nursing actions are neither legal nor ethical.
Example: The nurses delivered treatment that seemed futile and was based on a possible misunderstanding by the parents.	To tell Baby Michael's parents that the prescribed treatment is causing their child needless pain and they should stop all treatment.

Selection 4-4: "Caring for Pediatric Patients with HIV: Personal Concern and Ethical Dilemmas"

Since there is a quiz over the article as a test of mastery, you may again want to paperclip those pages together to keep students from peeking. The article includes a research study, but it also provides a review of concepts introduced in the textbook chapter and reiterated in the reference book. Encourage students to notice that they have some familiarity with the author's ideas.

TESTING: There are four questions in the Unit Test that pertain to this article. The questions test knowledge of the authors' purpose, of the results of the literature review, the authors' organization of the results, and the authors' conclusion.

"Right Answers"
After Reading 2

GOAL: *Test recall of relevant information*
TECHNIQUE: *Answer test questions*

Article Quiz Answers

A. Matching

1. d	4. b	7. c
2. e	5. g	8. f
3. i	6. h	9. a

B. Completion

10. *Confidentiality* was not maintained when the nurse discussed one patient's condition with another patient.

11. A medication error breaks the principle of *nonmaleficence*. The patient can be harmed by receiving the wrong drug.

12. The nurse is being confronted with the principle of *veracity*. Does he/she tell the patient what he/she knows or withhold the information? Since the physician has the responsibility of telling patients about their conditions, the nurse is caught in a real dilemma.

13. The nurse must maintain the principle of *justice*. This patient has the right to the same quality of care as any other patient. To do less based on opinion about the accusation against him or his behavior, race, religion, politics, and so on is to allow bias to determine nursing care.

C. Essay

14. Did you consider some of these points?

The significance of this study is limited in that it expresses some areas of concern of nurses in one setting, but it does suggest issues for further study with a broader population.

The fact that the authors made the effort to assess their fellow nurses regarding a perceived area of concern was a strength. If they can do a study and report it in a professional journal, other nurses can develop research projects too! The project may also contribute to the dialog at the institution where it was conducted and at other institutions where the article was read. It might serve as an impetus for other nurses to discuss their concerns.

Among the suggestions for improvement of the study's design are the following:

Increase the number of participants.

Select participants from across the country (or at least from a larger area of the country such as a state or a region).

Include male/female questions in the demographic information.

Select or develop a research tool to evaluate certain common issues.

Continue to seek narrated comments from participants.

Selection 4-5: "When Language Is an Obstacle"

This article represents a complete change of pace. The emphasis is on legal rather than on ethical considerations, and the topic is language. Students will probably bring their own experiences to this article, and, again, you may have to play a role in helping students identify their own stereotypes.

Students are asked to make an informal outline as a guide to understanding and then to explore some of the ideas in the article through their own insights. You may want to help students locate the reference notes related to legal cases and point out how they are cited. Our students often do not understand the outcome of the case involving Filipino nurses. You may want to determine if your students are having trouble understanding this case.

TESTING: Four of the questions in the Unit Test include one about the author's assumptions about the topic, another about the purpose in using a court case, a third about tactics to increase communication, and a fourth about the author's conclusion.

"Right Answers"
After Reading 3

GOAL: Test recall of relevant information
TECHNIQUE: Answer possible test questions

Based on your own experiences and what you've learned from this article, write a response to this biased question: "Why do people come to this country to work when they can't speak English?"

Here's one person's response. Yours will certainly be different, but it might mention some of the same points.

> There are lots of reasons people come to this country to work even if they were not born speaking English. How about looking at the other side of the question: What would you do if the best jobs in your field and the most opportunity for your family were in a non-English-speaking country? If you were as brave as I think you are, you would move, look for work, and then start taking language classes. Even if you started learning a new language today, you'd probably have a long wait before your American accent disappeared. In the meantime, you'd be tempted to lapse into English with expatriate coworkers, you might have to use writing if people can't understand you in the new language, and you might need a translator in certain situations. So, how about giving a break to people who have come here to work and to earn greater opportunities for their families?

Unit 5: Stress

Phases: Before, During, and After Reading

This is a shorter unit and includes only three publications. It is designed to allow students to extend and integrate practice in all three phases of the reading process. The After Reading activities include tests and application questions. The topic of stress is one with which you and your students will certainly be familiar at this late date in the term, so you may find that it is applicable in more than a theoretical way.

Selection 5-1: "Stress"

This medical-surgical text chapter is typical of the nursing presentation of stress. To give students experience with selective reading, three objectives from a typical nursing syllabus are included. The outcome goal is to answer a take-home test with 78 percent accuracy. The test questions are based on information in the chapter, but they require synthesis and application rather than literal comprehension.

TESTING: The Final Exam contains five test questions over this unit. The three questions that come from this chapter include a question about the theory of stress with which Selye is associated, a question about the stages of the GAS, and a third question about the areas to be included in the assessment of stress.

"Right Answers"
After Reading 3

GOAL: Periodically test recall of relevant material
TECHNIQUE: Answer possible test questions

Take-Home Test Answers

1. *B* is the best answer because the body's defenses are mobilized in the alarm stage. The extra circulation to the deep muscles allowed the girl to jump out of the van's way quickly.

2. The pilot's injuries are severe, and the GAS has worked to protect him despite the hemorrhage. However, after the thirty-minute hemorrhage, his defenses are expended, and he is now entering the stage of exhaustion, *D*. Without prompt medical assistance, the pilot may die.

3. a. This is not the best answer because the person having surgery almost always is concerned about some aspect. To say this minimizes those concerns and leaves the patient to worry about it alone.

   b. Usually family members can support the patient and provide some distraction. This is not the best answer either.

   c. Explaining what will take place before, during, and after surgery helps relieve the patient when the explanation is in words that can be understood. If the patient knows what to expect, he/she will probably be less anxious. C is the best answer.

   d. The patient may want to speak with a minister, rabbi, or other religious adviser, but this is optional and available only if the patient wishes.

4. Identify each of these coping resources as occurring in the person (P) or occurring in the environment (E).

   __P__   problem-solving skills
   __E__   utilitarian resources
   __P__   positive beliefs
   __P__   social skills

Give an example of each of the coping resources listed above.

problem-solving skills

> Being able to think of alternatives, gathering relevant information, identifying the problem

utilitarian resources

> Having money or other financial resources, using instructional manuals, using the services of social agencies

positive beliefs

> Believing in yourself (self-efficacy), having spiritual beliefs that are supportive

social skills

> Being able to communicate with others effectively, being able to get along with others (compatibility)

5. Suggest both an emotion-regulating (E-R) and a problem-solving (P-S) coping response to each of these demands. (Your response may be different. The following are provided as examples.)

   a. being diagnosed with AIDS
      E-R: Talking with a loved one about your feelings
      P-S: Calling the AIDS Hotline for information

   b. being turned down for a job
      E-R: Going out to a movie—a comedy, preferably
      P-S: Visiting the campus Career Center to look at job postings

c. making an oral book report in class
  E-R: On the day before the report, spending some time imagining yourself making the book report in a calm, effective manner
  P-S: Asking a classmate to listen to your report, and then listening to the other's report

d. Being asked to stay late at your job even though you have a quiz the next day and need time to review
  E-R: Letting the boss know that you understand the problem, but you are not able to stay late this evening
  P-S: Offering to call a co-worker who might be willing to come in to replace you

e. Learning that you have just been awarded a scholarship
  E-R: Jumping up and down with delight
  P-S: Making sure you understand to whom to send thank-you note

f. Realizing that you have never read one of the chapters to be covered on tomorrow's exam
  E-R: Deep breathing exercises
  P-S: Preview the chapter, correlate the chapter objectives to your outcome objectives, and get to work!

Selection 5-2: "Stress and Anxiety"

Many students regard this as the most difficult article in the book. Certainly, it provides a type of "graduation exercise," helping students to see how their comprehension has improved and what areas remain for improvement.

Although Robinson's vocabulary is elevated and the concepts are densely packed, her article is very well organized, following clues the author includes in topic sentences. Furthermore, only part of the article relates to the course objectives, so selective readers can spend their time on only a few sections rather than on reading the entire article.

There is a ten-question test, which is to be taken after students have completed their own note-making. You might paperclip the test pages and then ask to see the students' notes before allowing them to complete the test. The test instructions include a suggestion that students answer the questions from memory and then check their notes for corrections before looking to you for "Right Answers." It's useful for students to learn to distinguish between test mistakes caused by faulty comprehension and those caused by poor retention of correctly understood material. The three-stage answering process helps students gain the information they need for this analysis.

TESTING: The one test question on the final exam from this article asks students to select the best summary of Robinson's article.

"Right Answers"
After Reading 2

GOAL: Test recall of relevant information
TECHNIQUE: Review notes without rereading the text; answer possible test questions

1. b. comes from the first paragraph on page 236
2. d. supported on page 236 under Biologic Response
3. a. comes from the same paragraph as question 2 but is on page 237
4. b. comes from the last line of the first paragraph of the subheading Nursing Research on SI, T and P, on page 239

5. c. can be supported on page 240, in the first paragraph of Implications for Nursing Research and Practice, the last line
6. a. is found on page 240
7. d. is supported by the fifth sentence in the fourth paragraph on page 240
8. b. is found on page 241
9. c. supported on page 240
10. d. is supported on page 241, in the last paragraph before the summary

Selection 5-3: "Analyzing Job Demands and Coping Techniques"

What a breeze this article will seem after the "Stress and Anxiety" article. The After Reading activities require students to interview others based on the questions asked by the authors of the article. Locating these three questions and making appropriate adjustments for new interviewing situations is challenging for students. It may be helpful to let students read the article before discussing the interviewing assignment. Giving students a weekend to do interviews also yields better results. The insights students gain from the analysis of the interviews are often impressive.

TESTING: The test question over this article asks about the author's main purpose.

Unit 6: Review and Practice in Critical Thinking

This series of questions about all the publications in *RSNAH* provides an excellent review in preparation for a comprehensive final exam. It may also function as an extension of the reading strategies provided with each publication.

If used for review, students can be asked to choose one or two questions from each unit to present to the class. One class period can be devoted to reports from one or two units. Sometimes the size of the class makes it desirable for the students to work in pairs or trios to pool their talents in planning a response that might include illustrations, computer-based presentations, and oral or written reports. Creativity is definitely in order, and students frequently surprise themselves (and us) in the way they deal with the questions.

32

Unit Tests and Process Tests for Units 2–5

A Note on the Tests

Two types of tests are included here. The Unit Tests include several multiple-choice items over each of the publications in Units 2–5. The questions over the last unit are included in the Final Exam, which also presents selected items, slightly revised, from the earlier unit tests. Our effort has been to make the questions challenging and relevant. They involve comprehension of main ideas and details, which, in general, have been the subject of an activity in the reading process guides. Students are occasionally asked to select the best paraphrase or summary of a selection. These test questions are also designed to give students practice in answering the type of item that is contained in standardized reading tests.

The second type of test is the Process Test. Again, there is one provided for each of Units 2–5. These tests ask students to read relatively short articles and to answer questions related to the particular phase of the process under study in that unit. In the Process Test for Unit 4 (focusing on the After Reading Process), students will need to take a copy of the article home to read before taking the test in class. In the other cases, the articles are short enough to allow students to read the article and answer the test questions in the span of a class period. The Process Test may be used as an "essay question" with the multiple-choice questions on the unit tests.

Name _____

UNIT 2 TEST

1. The author of "Introduction to Physical Therapy" is
   a. a woman who edits a professional journal on physical therapy.
   b. the executive director of the Physical Therapy Society of the United States and Canada.
   c. a man who frequently publishes in nursing and medical periodicals.
   d. a college professor of physical therapy whose parents emigrated from Italy.

2. The major sections of the "Model Definition of Physical Therapy for State Practice Acts" are listed in this order:
   a. examining, alleviating, preventing, and engaging in other activities.
   b. consulting, researching, modifying, and functioning.
   c. evaluating, functioning, debriding, and maintaining.
   d. promoting fitness, health, and quality of life.

3. According to the author of "Introduction to Physical Therapy," the three characteristics of a profession that are generally agreed upon are
   a. dedication, organization, accuracy.
   b. knowledge, social value, autonomy of judgment.
   c. baccalaureate degree or higher, referral from a physician, service to the public.
   d. commitment, standards, supervision.

4. The section of the textbook you should use to locate the chapter called "Physical Therapy for the Older Adult" is the
   a. glossary.
   b. table of contents.
   c. index.
   d. title page.

5. "The Birth of a New Profession" by Cullinan and Cullinan is written by
   a. professional writers who have learned a great deal about radiology.
   b. retired radiologic technologists who know their subject first-hand.
   c. co-directors of the American Society of Radiologic Technologists.
   d. people who are too young to have any idea about the history of radiology.

6. The authors credit Elizabeth Fleischman Ascheim with
   a. the invention of x-rays.
   b. using x-rays to detect the accurate fit of shoes.
   c. being a pioneer who influenced the future of the profession.
   d. using x-rays to diagnose lung and heart conditions.

7. In the history of radiologic technologists, World Wars I and II
   a. resulted in the deaths of hundreds of technicians.
   b. created a backlash against technical equipment.
   c. made the need for identifying insignia evident.
   d. led to increased numbers of employees in radiography.

8. The transition to "a radiologic technologist" was largely completed by the
   a. 1960s.
   b. 1940s.
   c. 1920s.
   d. 1900s.

9. In her foreword to Leah Curtin's book, Margretta Madden Styles refers to the author as a
   a. nursing manager who knows how to crack the whip.
   b. dilettante who skims the surface of a vast pond.
   c. fine writer, pundit, and sage.
   d. collector who never throws anything away.

10. Curtin suggests that nurses, like ocean liners, need
    a. fog horns to warn others of their approach.
    b. to resist becoming rusty and obsolete.
    c. gyroscopes to maintain balance and perspective.
    d. goals that are clear and easy to follow.

11. Among the 1905 "Rules for Nurses" are
    a. the saying "When it is not necessary to change, it is necessary not to change."
    b. a raise of five percent is an option after five months if the hospital can afford it.
    c. nurses shall not work more than eight hours per day, thus leaving adequate time for rest and courting.
    d. to record observations carefully, nurses must make their pens carefully, whittling the nibs to their individual tastes.

12. Which of the following is the best paraphrase of this marginal heading in Florence Nightingale's "Chattering Hopes and Advices": *Chattering hopes the bane of the sick*?
    a. Making light of the dangers of a person's illness is very destructive to the sick.
    b. Sick people may chatter when they are fearful or chilled.
    c. Chatting with the sick may help them to become more hopeful.
    d. Ruining the hopes for recovery of a patient is an unethical act.

13. In understanding the times in which Nightingale lived and worked, it is helpful to realize that
    a. her contributions to nursing included high ethical standards and a concern for hygiene.
    b. she was among the first to recommend treatment with antibiotics.
    c. her membership in the British Women's Army Corps during the Crimean War was history-making.
    d. hypochondria was unknown during her lifetime.

14. Among the suggestions that Nightingale makes for pleasing sick people is that
    a. they should have private rooms because the air in the sick room could spread disease.
    b. babies make poor visitors for cheering up a patient because they often cry.
    c. patients should avoid caring for their pets because of the risk of exhaustion.
    d. visitors should share both their anxieties and good news.

15. One piece of advice that seems wrong in light of our current understanding of how disease is spread would be
    a. patients enjoy visitors who are lachrymose.
    b. the "air of the sick room" is no worse for babies than patients.
    c. some women admired for their pluck have brought ill health on themselves.
    d. vegetating is an effective way to avoid ill health.

16. Which of these terms might best be used to locate information on this learning objective: *Recognize principles of learning and the effect of each on health teaching.*
    a. client, patient, illness
    b. teaching, education, nursing
    c. learning, rules, effects
    d. communications, health promotion, teaching aids

17. According to Charlene Douglas in "Cultural Considerations for the African-American Population," acknowledging and appreciating cultural differences as well as making a sincere effort to understand the cultural context of a client's behavior are characteristic of
    a. a culturally competent nurse.
    b. culturally diverse populations.
    c. nurses just starting their careers.
    d. culturally prescribed patterns.

18. According to Douglas, the health efforts that will make the greatest strides in closing the disparity between health outcomes are
    a. never using first names in clinical settings, monitoring nonverbal communications, and not expecting eye contact.
    b. culturally sensitive, well developed, and well placed health education efforts.
    c. finding cures for AIDS, hypertension, and infant mortality.
    d. changing high-fat diets, lowering heart disease, and extending visitation privileges beyond immediate family.

19. In her article "Cultural Considerations: Asian-Americans and Pacific Islanders," Kem Louie indicated that
    a. there are unusual similarities among all the various groups making up this classification.
    b. AAPIs must be made to understand that the use of herbs and acupuncture is to be avoided.
    c. almost 100 percent of the AAPIs speak English.
    d. cigarette smoking is a health risk for these five groups.

20. Louie discusses access, availability, mental health, and utilization among the
    a. problems faced by Southeast Asian refugees.
    b. traditional health belief practices.
    c. implications for nursing interventions.
    d. health status profiles of monolinguals.

Reading and Remembering Process Test One

Phase 1, Before Reading

NOTE: None of the questions below asks you to read or write about the content of the attached article. Rather, the questions should reflect your understanding of the first phase of the reading process.

1. What are the goals of the first phase of the reading process: Before Reading?

2. One of the techniques useful in meeting Before-Reading goals is to preview a new assignment. Imagine that you have been asked to read the attached article, "Tomorrow's LPN: Understanding the Role," from *Nursing97*. List the features you would look at during a preview of this article. Your answer should include *specific* reference to this article. For example, if you recommend looking at the topic sentence, list the exact sentence you have in mind from the article.

3. Explain what you would expect to learn from looking at the features. In other words, what do you expect to know about an article before you begin to read it?

Career trends

Health care reform means

shifting career paths for

LPNs as well as RNs.

Whether you're an LPN or

an RN, you need to

understand where LPNs

are headed. Here are

answers to some crucial

questions.

Tomorrow's LPN: Understanding the Role

BY BETTY H. HUNT, LPN
President

MARY K. JAMES, LPN/DT
First Vice-President

National Federation of Licensed Practical Nurses, Inc.
Garner, N.C.

Q   How have the LPN role and scope of practice changed over the past few years?

A   Although the LPN role differs from state to state and from facility to facility, most LPNs are still employed as they always were—as health care team members working with the RN and physician. But some LPNs are now getting advanced preparation and taking positions in such areas as intravenous (I.V.) therapy, emergency medicine, and dialysis. They're also practicing in such settings as the intensive care unit, coronary care unit, and operating room. In these settings, they have to understand electrocardiograms, emergency drugs, cardiac medications, advanced assessment, and so forth.

Because of reductions in hospital staff, more LPNs are working in home health care, neighborhood health clinics, and insurance firms, where they investigate injuries and arrange for care and coverage. In nursing homes, many LPNs are now in leadership or charge positions, with the certified nursing assistant as the primary caregiver.

Q   How has LPN education changed?

A   As state boards of nursing reevaluate LPNs' scope of practice, the LPN curriculum changes to keep pace. For example, in some regions, the education program for LPNs is still only 8 months. In others, it's a year, and in at least one, it's 2 years.

Of course, education doesn't stop after graduation. For example, 24 states require continuing education for relicensure, according to a 1994 survey of the National Council of State Boards of Nursing, Inc.

Q   As an LPN, how should I prepare for the future?

A Here's what you'll need to do:

- *Keep learning.* You can't be part of the changes in health care if you're not willing to learn about them. Be sure you attend continuing-education seminars or classes. Make a point of upgrading your skills by getting advanced preparation in such skills as I.V. therapy, emergency medicine, or computer use in nursing.
- *Boost your career-building skills and attitudes.* These include thorough preparation for tasks, flexibility, and enthusiasm for new projects. Understand and get involved with the changes in health care delivery.
- *Network.* Connect to others and to your work. That means:
  - seeking out information about your profession locally and nationally
  - knowing your local, state, and national government representatives
  - participating in meetings where LPNs' work is a topic of discussion
  - learning who makes rulings and establishes policies about LPNs' work, such as members of your state board of nursing
  - seeking out support for your work from people both inside and outside health care, including consumers and educators
  - joining professional organizations, such as the National Federation of Licensed Practical Nurses, Inc.

By understanding the forces transforming health care and adapting to them, LPNs will continue to make up a crucial part of the health care system. Ultimately, that means reaching the same goal as RNs and other health care professionals: quality patient care.

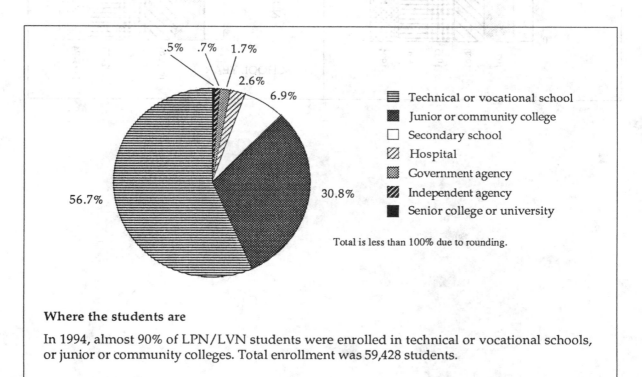

Where the students are

In 1994, almost 90% of LPN/LVN students were enrolled in technical or vocational schools, or junior or community colleges. Total enrollment was 59,428 students.

Source: *Nursing Datasource 1995*, National League for Nursing, New York.

Copyright © Houghton Mifflin Company. All rights reserved.

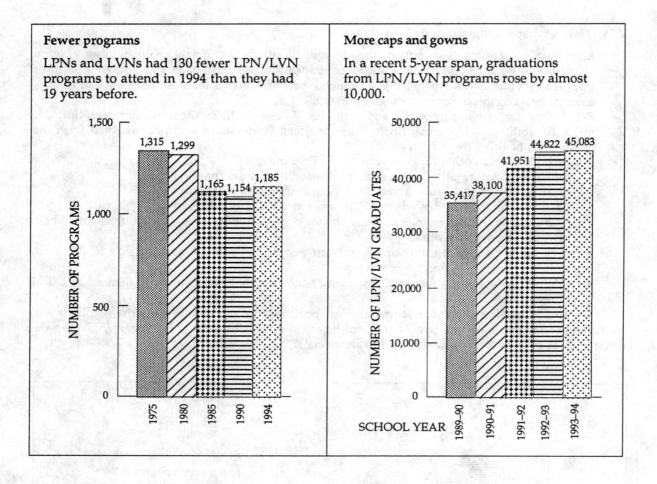

Fewer programs

LPNs and LVNs had 130 fewer LPN/LVN programs to attend in 1994 than they had 19 years before.

NUMBER OF PROGRAMS

1,315 1,299 1,165 1,154 1,185

1975 1980 1985 1990 1994

More caps and gowns

In a recent 5-year span, graduations from LPN/LVN programs rose by almost 10,000.

NUMBER OF LPN/LVN GRADUATES

35,417 38,100 41,951 44,822 45,083

SCHOOL YEAR

1989–90 1990–91 1991–92 1992–93 1993–94

Unit 2 Answer Key

1.	d	11.	d
2.	a	12.	a
3.	b	13.	a
4.	b	14.	d
5.	b	15.	b
6.	c	16.	c
7.	d	17.	a
8.	a	18.	b
9.	c	19.	d
10.	c	20.	c

Scoring Guide for Reading and Remembering Process Test One

1. Goals: Get oriented to the text, the author, the assignment, and the scope and organization of the information.

2. Preview: Title, authors and their roles in their North Carolina company, the introductory boxed print under the series title "Career trends," Q and A format (maybe reading the first exchange), the last paragraph (By understanding . . . quality patient care), and the three graphs.

3. By previewing the above, a reader would expect to discover that the authors are chief officers in a national organization for LPNs and that they have written a short article that is illustrated with three graphs and describes changes in the LPN career path.

Name _____

UNIT 3 TEST

1. In "Care of Patients with Pain," the author defines pain as
   a. a feeling of distress, suffering, or agony that is caused by stimulation of specialized nerve endings.
   b. a specific, individualized symptom of some diseases and injuries.
   c. whatever the person who is experiencing it says it is.
   d. a and c only.

2. The author supports her assertion that "the assumption that a person gets used to having continued pain simply is not true" with which of the following?
   a. Pain receptors are free nerve endings specially designed for their function.
   b. Pain receptors are abundantly distributed throughout the body.
   c. Unlike other types of receptors, pain receptors do not adapt or become less sensitive to repeated stimulation.
   d. The thalamus can only recognize an impulse as uncomfortable or disagreeable.

3. According to Melzak and Wall's Gate Control Theory of pain,
   a. signals for touch and pressure travel along larger nerve fibers than pain signals and may compete for passage through the gate.
   b. if two or more impulses arrive at the same gate at the same time, the pain impulse will prevail.
   c. massage, contrastimulation, acupressure, and other noninvasive techniques soothe pain signals before they arrive at a gate.
   d. the thalamus sorts through the various stimuli and decides which ones will be perceived as painful.

4. Location, quality, intensity, onset and precipitating factors, and measures that bring relief
   a. are among the myths that must be discarded when approaching patients' pain.
   b. constitute "proof" that a patient does or does not have pain.
   c. are key issues in determining whether a patient has chronic or acute pain.
   d. are among the subjective data that nurses gather in an effort to evaluate pain accurately.

5. Interventions such as combining tranquilizers, antidepressants, and narcotics; relaxation techniques; and biofeedback are interventions that would be most effective for patients with
   a. referred pain.
   b. ongoing or chronic pain.
   c. psychological pain.
   d. short-term or acute pain.

6. In "Nurses Plunged Me Into the Pain Cycle; Nurses Pulled Me Out," the author
   a. writes from personal experience.
   b. conducts research on the pain cycle.
   c. is a teacher who specializes in the topic of pain.
   d. has been the victim of surgical malpractice.

7. The author's primary purpose in the article is to
   a. narrate the sequence of events that led to her recovery.
   b. classify the types of pain treatment.
   c. illustrate the cause/effect relationship between anxiety and pain.
   d. compare and contrast pain treatment in two different facilities.

8. Which of the following is an example of *empathy* according to the nursing definition of the term?
   a. While she prepares to give an injection, a nurse shares her distress over her patient's pain.
   b. Feeling the patient's pain very strongly, a nurse refuses to administer any more intraspinal medication.
   c. Because the patient reacts stoically to pain, the nurse recognizes the patient's cultural background and suggests a milder form of medication.
   d. Even though the patient seems to be improving steadily, the nurse consistently delivers the prescribed pain medication on time.

9. The author concludes that "confidence makes the difference," which suggests that the
   a. nurses' lack of confidence in their ability to help caused her to have pain.
   b. nurses' reliability led to trust and greater participation in pain management.
   c. first hospital lacked confidence that she could recover.
   d. second hospital believed that patients could recover without medication if they had enough self-confidence.

10. In "Nurses' Judgments of Pain in Term and Preterm Newborns," the author's objective is to
    a. review the literature related to premature and full-term babies' pain.
    b. show nurses videotapes of newborns in pain, so they will recognize newborns' distress next time.
    c. prove that the pain of preterm newborns is misassessed.
    d. examine judgments of pain intensity and cues used by nurses in assessing pain.

11. The author reports results indicating that
    a. nurses think that preterm newborns experience more pain than full-term newborns.
    b. nurses rated the pain intensity higher for full-term newborns whom they saw on videotape.
    c. in some cases, the cues nurses use to assess newborns' pain reveal a high level of sympathy for preterm newborns.
    d. previously reported research showed a different set of cues to assess pain than the ones used in this study.

12. The best summary of the "Discussion and Nursing Implications" section is which of the following?
    a. The misperception of preterm newborns' pain could have significant consequences for the neonate. Since experience didn't make a difference in the recognition of neonatal pain, the study suggests that nurses need continuing education about pain assessment in newborns.
    b. Short-term pain may affect newborns' activities, and ongoing pain can lead to greater susceptibility to illness. Thus, continuing education in the neurobehavioral development of newborns is needed.
    c. Since there were statistically significant differences in the pain ratings for preterm and full-term newborns, nurses' training should include practice in the rating of neonates' pain. They should learn more sophisticated cues than "turned red in the face."
    d. The study should be repeated in other hospitals and with other assessment instruments to determine whether bias in the methodology or population accounts for the results.

13. In "Review of Literature on Culture and Pain of Adults, with Focus on Mexican-Americans," the authors
    a. conducted an experiment involving Mexican-American adults.
    b. reviewed literature that included Mexican-Americans' beliefs about pain.
    c. concluded that Mexican-Americans are complainers who want immediate relief for their pain.
    d. made recommendations for increasing pain medication for Mexican-Americans in view of their reluctance to ask for it.

14. The Zborowski study reports that
    a. cultural traditions determine if and when a person experiences pain.
    b. moaning and crying should always be interpreted as signs of pain.
    c. all individuals respond to pain in essentially the same ways.
    d. hospital staff tend to reflect "Old American" responses to pain.

15. According to one study mentioned in the article, crying, moaning, and stoicism
    a. are characteristic ways of responding to Mexican-American patients.
    b. are typical "Yankee" responses to pain.
    c. might function one way among Mexican-American patients and another way among "Old Americans."
    d. are examples of inappropriate behaviors.

16. The authors see which of the following implications for transcultural nursing practice?
    a. Nursing pain assessments should investigate the meaning a patient attaches to particular pain behaviors and the type of intervention desired by the patient.
    b. The extent to which a patient holds traditional beliefs should be the subject of further research.
    c. Quantitative research is needed to explore cultural beliefs.
    d. Pain assessment tools are not used frequently enough in current nursing practice.

17. In "Avoiding Opioid-Induced Respiratory Depression," the authors define clinically significant respiratory depression as a(n)
    a. clinically defined level of respirations below 10 per minute when the patient is resting.
    b. frequent occurrence in hospitalized patients resulting from the severity of their illness.
    c. desirable precursor to complete sedation with the use of narcotics.
    d. event which requires intervention to reverse it and prevent progression to respiratory arrest.

18. Among the risk factors for opioid-induced respiratory depression are
    a. pulse, blood pressure, and adventitious sounds.
    b. age, renal dysfunction, and opioid tolerance.
    c. history with opioids, concurrent medications, and opioid naiveté.
    d. dosages above 300 mg, postoperative medications, and aged under 10 or over 50.

19. The best way to monitor the sedation level and respiratory status according to the authors is for the
    a. nurse to anticipate the patient's pain.
    b. nurse to observe the patient's breathing and sedation.
    c. patient to stay alert and ask for no more medication than is absolutely necessary to relieve pain.
    d. patient to use an instrument called a pulse oximeter.

20. The sedation level of a patient who can neither complete a sentence nor respond to a request to do prescribed exercises without falling asleep would be ranked as
    a. 1 = awake and alert.
    b. 2 = occasionally drowsy, easy to arouse.
    c. 3 = frequently drowsy, arousable, drifts off to sleep during conversation.
    d. 4 = somnolent, minimal or no response to stimuli.

Reading and Remembering Process Test Two

Phase 2, During Reading

1. What are the goals of the second phase of the reading process: During Reading?

2. One of the techniques applied During Reading is to use your understanding of main ideas and paragraph organization. To demonstrate your mastery of that technique, answer the following questions about the attached article, "Pain Management Handbook," from *Nursing97*.

    a. How many main sections are there in the body of this article (excluding graphics)?

    b. What is the main idea of the first section in the article? (Choose a sentence from the article or construct a main idea sentence of your own to write in this space.)

c. What is the main idea of the last section in the article? (Choose a sentence from the article or construct a main idea sentence of your own to write in this space.)

d. What organizational pattern does the author use to develop the first and the last sections of the article?

Pain Management
HANDBOOK:

Practical tips for relieving your patient's pain

MARGO MCCAFFERY, RN, MS, FAAN
Nursing Consultant • Pain Management • Los Angeles, Calif.

Assessing sedation

Sedation precedes opioid-induced respiratory depression. To prevent opioid-induced respiratory depression, assess the patient's sedation level at regular intervals (every 1 to 2 hours for the first 8 to 12 hours). Assess all patients who are receiving opioids via intramuscular, intravenous, or spinal routes to relieve moderate to severe pain and who haven't been on regular doses of opioids. Here's an example of a sedation scale along with nursing interventions:

S = sleeping; easily aroused; requires no action
1 = awake and alert; requires no action
2 = occasionally drowsy; easy to arouse; requires no action
3 = frequently drowsy; arousable; drifts off to sleep during conversation. Decrease the opioid dose.
4 = somnolent; minimal or no response to stimuli. Discontinue opioid and consider use of naloxone (Narcan).

Using naloxone

When a patient suffers respiratory depression from an opioid prescribed for analgesia, physical stimulation and discontinuing the opioid may arouse him.

But if the patient doesn't respond to instructions to take a deep breath, use an opioid antagonist, such as naloxone (Narcan), to quickly reverse potentially fatal opioid-induced respiratory arrest. Titrate naloxone to the patient's response: If you give too much naloxone or give it too quickly, you'll also reverse analgesia. Follow these steps.

1. Evaluate the patient. Patients receiving opioids for analgesia who require naloxone usually:
   • are unresponsive to physical stimulation
   • have shallow respirations or a respiratory rate less than seven breaths per minute
   • have recently received an opioid dose
   • have pinpoint pupils

Comparing analgesics

These doses of oral analgesics are approximately equivalent when used for mild to moderate pain.

Analgesic	P.O. dose
Nonopioids	
Acetaminophen (Tylenol)	650 mg
Aspirin	650 mg
Opioids	
Codeine	30–60 mg
Meperidine (Demerol)	50 mg
Pentazocine HCl (Talwin)	30–50 mg
Propoxyphene HCl (Darvon)	65 mg
Propoxyphene napsylate (Darvon-N)	100 mg

Source: *Principles of Analgesic Use in the Treatment of Acute Pain and Cancer Pain,* 3rd edition, Skokie, Ill., American Pain Society, 1992.

Reevaluate if the patient doesn't meet these criteria or has been receiving opioids for a week or longer. Patients on long-term opioid therapy develop a physical tolerance so they're less likely to experience opioid-induced respiratory depression.

2. Discontinue the opioid and any other sedative drugs, but maintain intravenous (I.V.) access.
3. Call for help. Ask a colleague to bring naloxone to the bedside. Remain with the patient and continue trying to arouse him.
4. Mix 0.4 mg of naloxone and 10 ml of 0.9% sodium chloride solution in a syringe for I.V. administration. (If you can't access the I.V. route, administer 0.4 mg of undiluted naloxone subcutaneously or intramuscularly.)
5. Administer the dilute naloxone solution by I.V. push slowly (0.5 ml every 2 minutes) while you closely observe the patient's response. Titrate to effect.
   Note: This dosage is less than that typically given to a patient with respiratory depression or arrest of unknown cause (for example, an unconscious patient brought into the emergency department with a suspected opioid overdose).
6. The patient should open his eyes and talk within 1 to 2 minutes. If he doesn't, continue giving I.V. naloxone at the same rate to a maximum of 0.8 mg or 20 ml of dilute naloxone. If he still doesn't respond, look for other causes of sedation and respiratory depression.
7. As soon as the patient is alert and breathing at nine or more breaths per minute, discontinue the naloxone, but keep the syringe at the bedside. Because the duration of naloxone is shorter than that of most opioids, he may need another dose of naloxone as early as 30 minutes after the first dose.
8. Monitor the patient's sedation and respiratory status and encourage him to take deep breaths every 1 to 2 minutes until he's more alert.
9. Notify the patient's physician, and document your actions.
10. Provide nonopioid pain relief (for example, a nonsteroidal anti-inflammatory drug) as prescribed, to reduce the amount of opioid needed to control pain.
11. Resume opioid administration at half the original dose, as prescribed, when the patient is easily aroused and his respiratory rate is greater than nine breaths per minute.

Opioids and the elderly

If you'll be administering an opioid to your elderly patient, remember these points:

- Elderly patients may experience a higher peak effect and longer duration of pain relief from an opioid. Start with 25% to 50% of the recommended adult dose and titrate upward slowly as needed.
- Increase doses in elderly patients based on *patient response* (comfort and adverse reactions) rather than a preconceived notion of what the patient "should" require.
- Meperidine (Demerol) is the least-desirable opioid choice for elderly patients. Its metabolite, normeperidine, can accumulate in elderly patients with impaired renal function and cause serious central nervous system excitation, such as twitching, jerking, and having seizures.

Rating the basic pain measures

When assessing your patient's level of pain, follow these pain-rating guidelines, listed in descending order of importance. Whenever available, use a patient's self-report of pain.

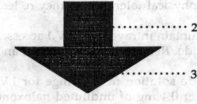

Most important............ 1. Patient's self-report

.... 2. Report of parent, family member, or others close to the patient

.... 3. Behaviors (for example, facial expressions, body movements, crying)

Least important........... 4. Physiologic measures

Getting a jump on pain

When treating pain that is present most of the day:

- DO consider implementing p.r.n. analgesic orders around-the-clock if your patient has pain 12 or more hours out of 24.
- DO wake the patient and give him pain medication before the pain wakes him.
- DO teach the patient to request pain medication before pain occurs (if he can predict it) or as soon as pain occurs and before it increases.

Three addiction don'ts

Remember these three points when you suspect that your patient is addicted to drugs.

1. DON'T label a patient as an addict. A diagnosis of addiction requires careful assessment.
2. DON'T assume that a patient seeking pain relief is seeking drugs.
3. DON'T allow biases about addiction to interfere with providing the best possible pain relief for the addicted patient.

Classifying analgesics: Keep these categories in mind

Nonopioids

- *Acetaminophen* (Tylenol)
- *NSAIDs:*
aspirin, ibuprofen (Advil, Nuprin), ketorolac (Toradol), naproxen (Naprosyn), naproxen sodium (Aleve), piroxicam (Feldene)

Opioids

- *Mu-agonists (full agonists):* codeine (as in Tylenol No. 3), fentanyl (Duragesic patch), hydrocodone (Vicodin), hydromorphone (Dilaudid), meperidine (Demerol), oxycodone (as in Percocet, Tylox)

- *Agonist-antagonists:* pentazocine HCl (Talwin), butorphanol (Stadol)

Adjuvants

- *Multipurpose:* dexamethasone (Decadron), dextroamphetamine (Dexadrine), methylphenidate (Ritalin)

- *Tricyclic antidepressants:* amitryptiline (Elavil), desipramine (Norpramin), imipramine (Tofranil)

- *Anticonvulsants* carbamazepine (Tegretol), clonazepam (Klonopin), phenytoin (Dilantin)

Which analgesic groups can be combined?

May be useful

- Acetaminophen + NSAID: Combining acetaminophen with any of the NSAIDs may add analgesia without increasing adverse effects.

- Opioid + nonopioid: Even if pain is severe enough to require an opioid, the addition of acetaminophen or an NSAID should be considered.

- Adjuvant + opioid + nonopioid: Appropriate for chronic pain

Not recommended

- NSAID + NSAID: Adds little additional pain relief and the risk of adverse effects is considerable.

- Mu-agonist + agonist-antagonist: This combination may reverse analgesia of the mu-agonist or precipitate withdrawal in a physically dependent patient.

- Mu-agonist + mu-agonist: Complicates treatment with little or no advantage; adverse effects are additive.

Source: McCaffery, M.: "Analgesics: Mapping Out Pain Relief." *Nursing96*. January, 41–46.

Quick list: Pain resources

American Alliance of Cancer Pain Initiatives
The Resource Center
1300 University Ave.
Room 4720
Madison, WI 53706
(608) 265-4013

American Chronic Pain Association
P.O. Box 850
Rocklin, CA 95677
(916) 632-0922

American Pain Society
4700 W. Lake Ave.
Glenview, IL 60025
(847) 375-4715

American Society of Pain Management Nurses
2755 Bristol Street
Suite 110
Costa Mesa, CA 92628
(714) 545-1305

Mayday Pain Resources Center
City of Hope Medical Center
1500 E. Duarte Rd.
Duarte, CA 91010
(818) 359-8111, ext. 3829

Unit 3 Answer Key

1.	d	11.	b
2.	c	12.	a
3.	a	13.	b
4.	d	14.	d
5.	b	15.	c
6.	a	16.	a
7.	d	17.	d
8.	d	18.	c
9.	b	19.	b
10.	d	20.	c

Scoring Guide for Reading and Remembering Process Test Two

1. Goals: Monitor comprehension and achievement of purpose.

2. a. Main sections: There are five headings in the article (with an additional six or seven in the graphics).

   b. Main idea of the first section (constructed sentence): Assess the sedation level of most patients taking opioids by using a 4-point scale.

      (The first sentence isn't an effective statement of the main idea in the first section because it doesn't cover most of the ideas in the paragraph. The second sentence might be acceptable, but it doesn't cover the rating scale, which makes up a large part of the section.)

   c. Main idea of the last section, "Three Addiction Don'ts" (constructed sentence): Nurses who suspect their patients are addicts shouldn't label them, make assumptions about their seeking drugs, or allow bias to keep them from providing effective pain relief.

      (The main idea statement should contain at least the flavor of the three don'ts, rather than just stating that there are three points to be remembered.)

   d. The author uses listing in both sections.

Name _____

UNIT 4 TEST

1. According to Kozier and Erb in "Ethics and Values," the term that stands for an activity, beliefs, and expected standards is
   a. ethnicity.
   b. law.
   c. ethics.
   d. values.

2. The authors define *moral dilemmas* as involving
   a. a clear conflict of two or more moral principles.
   b. cognitive moral development.
   c. bioethics.
   d. a morals problem.

3. Moral rules are built upon moral principles that include
   a. social movements and technology.
   b. value systems and purposive behavior.
   c. decision-focused and action-focused problems.
   d. beneficence and veracity.

4. "The Golden Rule" provides a good example of
   a. teleological decision making.
   b. deontology.
   c. moral theories.
   d. intuitionism.

5. When a nurse participates in his or her own continuing education by reading a journal article, answering the questions provided, and sending them in to be graded, the nurse is exhibiting
   a. moral behavior.
   b. support for the ANA's Code for Nurses.
   c. respect for persons.
   d. conflicting loyalties.

6. In "Ethical Perceptions of Parents and Nurses in NICU: The Case of Baby Michael," the authors identify which of the following issues of concern to both parents and nurses?
   a. Treatment, informed consent, and decision making
   b. Disconnection from infant, withdrawal of treatment, and inadequate disclosure of information
   c. Crisis intervention, caring processes, and ethical dilemmas
   d. Negligence, duty to act, and liability

7. Nurses are encouraged to listen to parents tell and retell stories in order to
   a. reopen a social world.
   b. explore coping mechanisms.
   c. gain an intellectual understanding of the crisis.
   d. help bring present feelings into the open.

8. The case of Baby Michael provided the following details:
   a. Baby Michael was born at 52 weeks following a cesarean section performed when he was in fetal distress. As a result, he experienced cardiac arrest. His parents agreed to a DNR (do not resuscitate) order, but the baby survived on his own. He was able to leave the hospital, but the brain damage he had experienced made it hard for him to breathe or suck.

   b. Baby Michael was born at eight months, following his mother's uncontrollable uterine contractions. He was placed on a ventilator which led to a pneumothorax. The treatment for this condition was painful, but the parents seemed unaware of his pain. They took the baby home before hospital personnel recommended his release.

   c. Baby Michael was born prematurely and received standard treatment. When he developed infections and had other severe problems, the parents asked for every possible effort to save his life. The baby left the hospital several months later when he was able to breathe on his own and nurse.

   d. Baby Michael was born at six months, three years after his mother's first pregnancy. He was treated for Grade III intracranial bleeding and other problems, which the nursing staff thought were unnecessary and excessive. However, he was able to leave the hospital having achieved age-appropriate neuromuscular development.

9. Which of the following is the best paraphrase of this sentence, "In summary, the NICU environment is fraught with ethical dilemmas, as evidenced by the cited studies"?
   a. Finally, the environment for neonates has become filled with moral decisions as the studies you see prove.
   b. In short, the studies we have included show that the NICU is filled with difficult moral choices.
   c. A summary of the literature shows that there are many moral syllogisms in NICUs.
   d. There are many ethical dilemmas in the NICU environment as evidenced by the cited studies.

10. In "Ethical Decision Making," four types of situations with varying relationships between ethics and the law are presented:
    Type 1: actions are both ethical and legal
    Type 2: actions may be considered ethical but not legal
    Type 3: actions may be considered legal but not ethical
    Type 4: actions are neither legal nor ethical
    Which of these types are labeled "ambiguous"?
    a. Types 1 and 2
    b. Types 2 and 3
    c. Types 3 and 4
    d. Types 1 and 4

11. The article outlines various categories of decisions. Which decision would apply to the following situation?
    A student is confronted with a decision about whether to report having seen a classmate cheat on a test. The student decides to wait to find out whether the classmate has passed the test.
    a. Active decision
    b. Passive decision
    c. Programmed decision
    d. Nonprogrammed decision

12. Which ethical theory forms the basis of this decision?
    a. Moral relativism
    b. Teleology
    c. Deontology
    d. Intuitionism

13. According to the text, if everyone practiced _____, the following would occur: There would be no objective way to resolve moral dilemmas, a person could not question another's moral judgment, professional standards would become meaningless, and law and order in society would disappear.
    a. Moral relativism
    b. Teleology
    c. Deontology
    d. Intuitionism

14. In "Caring for Pediatric Patients with HIV," Murphy and Famolare's purpose was to
    a. use direct quotes from nurses to illustrate ethical decision making.
    b. review literature on ethics relating to care of children with HIV.
    c. conduct formal research into nursing dilemmas.
    d. raise questions and show common dilemmas for the nurses surveyed.

15. As they looked through the available research articles, the authors discovered
    a. that only a few studies were relevant to their survey.
    b. many studies that replicated the work they did.
    c. a discrepancy between their survey results and others'.
    d. that the ANA has no statement of ethics related to patients with HIV.

16. The authors organized their survey results according to
    a. the ANA Code's list of ethical perspectives.
    b. the themes revealed by the literature.
    c. ethical and legal principles specifically applicable to health care.
    d. medicolegal concepts.

17. The authors conclude that HIV-related ethical dilemmas are distinctive because
    a. professional and personal concerns become inseparable.
    b. no other disease is so frightening.
    c. their survey proved that most nurses have similar concerns.
    d. there has been so much discussion of the issue in the press.

18. In the article "When Language Is an Obstacle," Sloan assumes that
    a. all nurses speak English.
    b. a diversity of languages only enriches the workplace.
    c. knowing the legal basis for on-the-job communication can have several benefits.
    d. patients who don't speak English are someone else's responsibility.

19. A court case is used to illustrate which of the following issues?
    a. The EEOC maintains that an individual's primary language is an essential characteristic of national origin.
    b. Legitimate business needs include efficiency, productivity, and order.
    c. Strict English-only rules in the workplace that prohibit workers from speaking a foreign language even while on breaks or at lunch are likely to violate the civil rights of employees.
    d. Some on-duty language restrictions are acceptable if they are motivated by a concern for patient safety.

20. According to the article, using faxes, computers, and written confirmation are tactics that can help which situation?
    a. The non-English-speaking patient has a relative in another city who speaks English well.
    b. The nurse feels that a consultant is necessary to interpret the doctor's orders.
    c. The doctor's verbal orders are difficult to understand because of a heavy accent.
    d. The hospital wants confirmation of an unusual diagnosis made by a doctor educated in another country.

21. The author concludes with the idea that
    a. patients who don't speak English well really should take a course to improve their proficiency.
    b. when using a family member as a translator, it is inappropriate to request the patient's consent.
    c. learning about another culture may be rewarding both professionally and personally.
    d. the ADA protects speakers of other languages from discrimination.

Reading and Remembering Process Test Three

Phase 3, After Reading

NOTE: To prepare for this test, students should take the article on protecting patients' privacy home to read and mark a day or two before the test. In class, they will answer the following questions, using their marked copy of the article.

1. What are the goals of the third phase of the reading process: After Reading?

2. Answer the Continuing Education Test that appeared with the original article. Feel free to use your notes in deciding which answer to choose. When you choose an answer, mark the spot in the article on which you based your answer. In other words, there should be seven numbers in the margin of your article, one for each of the right answers on the test. Turn in both your marked article and these test pages when you have finished.

Continuing Education Test

1. The patient's right to have health information kept private is based on
   a. JCAHO standards.
   b. the ANA Code of Nurses.
   c. State Board of Nursing regulations.
   d. the U.S. Constitution.

2. The nurse who fails to report child abuse may be subject to a fine and
   a. immediate termination.
   b. disciplinary action.
   c. civil action.
   d. arrest.

3. Prior to faxing medical information, the sender must *first*
   a. check with the risk manager.
   b. get a written order from the physician.
   c. ask the patient to sign a consent form.
   d. verify there is an authorized person available to receive it.

4. Based on the Tarasoff case in California, which legal obligation for health care providers was established?
   a. Report all HIV cases
   b. Disclose information about a threat to a person's safety
   c. Document genetic test results in health care records
   d. Assure confidentiality of computerized records

5. Which patient information is generally *not* considered privileged?
   a. Diagnosis
   b. Prognosis
   c. Treatments ordered
   d. Admission and discharge dates

6. Nationwide, nurses are required to report which situation to the police?
   a. Rape
   b. Illicit drug use
   c. Pregnancy in minors
   d. Gunshot or stab wounds

7. Which states recently enacted laws that allow providers to notify police about the results of tests that show alcohol levels?
   a. Alabama and Texas
   b. Florida and Nebraska
   c. Illinois and Oregon
   d. New York and Pennsylvania

Protecting Patients' Privacy

GAYLE H. SULLIVAN, RN, JD

The author, a member of the *RN* editorial board, is president of
Quality Assurance Associates, Inc., a medical liability consulting firm
in Fairfield, Conn. She conducts legal seminars for nurses nationwide.

STAFF EDITOR: MARISSA J. VENTURA

Protecting the confidentiality of a patient's health information used to be as simple as securing his chart from unauthorized eyes and holding discussions with or about him out of earshot of those who did not provide direct care.

Today, it is much more problematic. State laws and court rulings have created a number of exceptions to general confidentiality requirements. Public concern over sensitive issues such as HIV and genetic test results has led to a debate about special protections to ensure patients' privacy. And, technology has increased the ways patient information can be shared and, therefore, the number of people who have access to it.

Every nurse, then, needs to know when and how to protect a patient's right to privacy—a right based on the U.S. Constitution and upheld by laws in all 50 states. Here's a look at the key issues and liability risks.

When are you compelled to disclose?

You have a legal duty to report certain situations in which the safety of the patient or the welfare of the public is considered at risk. Most jurisdictions require reporting of child and elder abuse and other illegal actions, situations in which the patient may harm another, and communicable diseases. Because reporting requirements vary by state, you'll need to check with your risk manager or local statutes for specific provisions in your jurisdiction.

In general, however, as long as you report in good faith and according to the law, most statutes provide immunity from civil and criminal liability. And failure to report could subject you to a fine and disciplinary action.

Here are the four main exceptions to the rule of patient-provider confidentiality:

Child and elder abuse. Every state requires nurses and physicians to report cases of suspected child abuse, neglect, and abandonment to the appropriate state agency or the police. A child is generally defined as anyone who is under the age of 18.

All states also require nurses in nursing homes to report cases of suspected elder abuse, neglect, and abandonment. Most states impose the same reporting requirement on nurses in other settings as well. The definition of an elderly patient varies—in Connecticut, for example, it's anyone who is over the age of 60—and some statutes don't specify an age.

Follow your employer's reporting policy. Document all observations of suspected abuse or neglect in the patient's chart, both physical (bruises, lesions, and so on) and psychological (fear or a withdrawn disposition).

Other criminal activity. All 50 states mandate that rape cases be reported to the police.[1] In some jurisdictions, narcotic use or evidence of violent crimes—such as gunshot or stab wounds—must be reported, as well.

Recently, Illinois and Oregon enacted laws that weaken the confidentiality rights of patients who are being treated for motor vehicle accident injuries. These states now allow health care providers to notify police about the results of blood or urine tests that show alcohol or drug levels above the legal limit. Maine has a similar law which states that if an RN or other provider knows or reasonably suspects that a patient who has been involved in a motor vehicle accident has been driving while under the influence of alcohol or drugs, she may report this to the police. So, nurses in these states who wish to report drivers who are drunk or high can do so without legal repercussions.

Dangerous patients. If a patient tells you that he is going to harm another person, you may be obligated to disclose that information to protect the intended victim. That duty was established more than 20 years ago with the landmark Tarasoff case, in which the California Supreme Court found a psychotherapist liable for failing to warn a woman of his patient's plan to kill her—a plan that was carried out.[2]

If your patient makes such a threat, document it in his chart—in quotes and in his exact words, if possible—and question him further. If you believe the threat has merit, immediately inform your supervisor, risk manager, or the physician so that appropriate actions can be taken to avert harm.

Communicable diseases. Certain infectious conditions must be reported to the appropriate state or local agency or health department. The most controversial disease on the reporting list: HIV/AIDS.

Every state requires the reporting of AIDS cases for epidemiological purposes—some require the reporting of the patient's name and address, while others prohibit the disclosure of any identifying data. Moreover, 28 states mandate the reporting—by name—of patients diagnosed with HIV. Some states also permit disclosure of a patient's HIV-positive status to third parties—say, a sexual partner or needle-sharing partner. However, many states allow only a physician or a public health officer—not the patient's nurse—to disclose this information. (See last month's Legally Speaking for more on HIV confidentiality parameters.)

When disclosure requires consent

Generally, informational data such as a patient's name, address, and dates of admission or discharge are not considered confidential information and therefore not protected by law. Information related to diagnosis, treatment, and prognosis, however, *is* considered confidential. Before disclosing this information to anyone other than members of the health care team—and unless otherwise mandated by law or a court order—you must obtain your patient's consent.

Verbal consent, either implicit or explicit, is usually sufficient to discuss your patient's health face-to-face with concerned family members or friends. You should try to avoid disclosing such information over the telephone, whenever possible. You never know who is really on the other end of the line.

But for anyone else—and especially when you're sending his actual medical records—obtain *written* authorization from the patient or, if he's unconscious, his representative.

In most cases, this can simply be a signed letter from the patient or a signed general consent form, such as the kind insurance companies use. In certain instances, however, a general letter or release is not enough.

Information related to a patient's HIV/AIDS status (other than that governed by the disclosure rules discussed earlier), psychiatric condition, and drug or alcohol treatment receives special protection from disclosure under federal and state laws. You are prohibited from releasing any such information—including the patient's name or dates of admission or discharge—without your patient's *specific* consent.

As with a general release form, a patient's specific consent must be in writing, dated, and signed by him or his proxy. It must also state the purpose of the disclosure, the specific data to be revealed, to whom it can be revealed, who can make the disclosure, and how long the consent is valid.

When you're sending specially protected health information through the mail, make sure that it's accompanied by a statement of confidentiality, which prohibits the receiving party from revealing the information without the patient's consent. If you're disclosing the information verbally, you are not duty bound to recite this statement—but it certainly wouldn't hurt.

Currently, no special cloak of protection exists for another sensitive type of health information—genetic test results. But that is likely to change as more and more patients are tested for genes that mutate to cancer and other diseases.

Genetic information has raised fears by patients that their employers will discriminate against them and that insurance companies will deny or limit coverage. Some women who carry genes linked to breast or ovarian cancer are asking their doctors not to include this information in their medical records. Some doctors are complying with these requests, relying instead on their memories and pretending not to know any genetic information when they are dealing with insurers and other physicians.[3]

It's a thorny issue—what to do if a patient asks you not to chart potentially explosive information pertaining to diagnosis, prognosis, or treatment. At this point, it remains largely an ethical call that each health care professional must make for him- or herself.

Technology brings legal pitfalls, too

Developments in communication technology have made the business of caring for patients more efficient. But using computers, fax machines, videotapes, and telephones to process, store, or transmit patient information has set the stage for security violations like never before.

Fortunately, the federal government has stepped in to help. The Health Insurance Portability and Accountability Act of 1996 mandates, among other things, that Congress establish privacy rules to manage electronic records within three and a half years of the law's enactment. These rules must stipulate that anyone with access to computerized health information be given training on maintaining confidentiality.

You should already be taking steps to ensure the privacy of electronic information. If you use a computer by the patient's bedside or at the nurses station, clear the screen after each use. Position the screen in a way that passersby cannot see it. And, don't give your password to anyone.

Be sure to keep videotapes and backup computer disks—as well as paper records—in a secure place for the amount of time required by law. Never reuse tapes or disks because they may not be completely erased.

Avoid faxing medical information whenever possible. If it's unavoidable, verify the number you'll be sending the fax to and determine in advance that an authorized party will be on hand to receive it as soon as it comes in.

When providing health information over the phone, do so in a private area. Always verify to whom you are speaking and whether that person is entitled to information about a patient's health. If the party you are calling is not in, don't leave a message that reveals anything about a patient's condition. Instead ask to have the party you are calling return the call.

Of course, many breaches of confidentiality have nothing to do with technology at all. They occur when providers discuss confidential data in areas where they can be overheard. Hold all such discussions in a private location, away from unauthorized ears. When talking to a patient who is not in a private room, remember to keep your voice down.

Trust is a cornerstone of the patient-provider relationship. Making sure your patient's health information stays confidential will help you uphold that trust. Understanding the exceptions to confidentiality rules in select situations will help put you on a course that's liability-free.

References

1. Greve, P. A. (1990). Keep quiet or speak up? Issues in patient confidentiality. *RN, 53*(12), 53.

2. Tarasoff v. The Regents of the University of California, 13 Cal. 3d 177, 529 P.2d 553 (1974).

3. Kolata, G. (1997, February 4). Advent of testing for breast cancer genes leads to fears of disclosure and discrimination. *The New York Times,* p. C1.

Unit 4 Answer Key

1.	c	12.	b
2.	a	13.	a
3.	d	14.	d
4.	b	15.	a
5.	b	16.	c
6.	a	17.	a
7.	d	18.	c
8.	c	19.	d
9.	b	20.	c
10.	b	21.	c
11.	b		

Scoring Guide for Reading and Remembering Process Test 3

1. The three goals are to check initial recall of relevant information, organize it for recall, and test recall of the relevant information periodically.

2. Continuing Education Test Answers

1.	d	4.	b	7.	c
2.	b	5.	d		
3.	d	6.	a		

Marking the Location of Right Answers

1. The answer to Question 1 is located in the last paragraph of the introduction, the third paragraph in the article. To us, the source of the right to privacy seemed a minor detail, so it wasn't marked.

2. The answer to Question 2 is located in the second paragraph of the heading "When are you compelled to disclose?" Again, it seemed like a minor detail (although it certainly wouldn't seem that way to a fined nurse!), so it wasn't underlined.

3. This answer is located in the last column of the article, the fourth paragraph from the end. It does seem like one of the two important ideas about faxing contained in the paragraph.

4. Question 4 is in the first paragraph of the "Dangerous patients" section. Although memorizing the name of the court case isn't important, this case is an important detail in the section.

5. This question is answered in the section "When disclosure requires consent." It requires specific details about the main idea.

6. Question 6 is answered in the first paragraph of "Other criminal activity." The right answer is a major detail.

7. The answer to this question is also in the "Other criminal activity" section, in the paragraph below the one about rape. It seems likely that readers from Illinois and Oregon would be more inclined to remember this detail than would those from other states.

Protecting Patients' Privacy

GAYLE H. SULLIVAN, RN, JD

The author, a member of the *RN* editorial board, is president of
Quality Assurance Associates, Inc., a medical liability consulting firm
in Fairfield, Conn. She conducts legal seminars for nurses nationwide.

STAFF EDITOR: MARISSA J. VENTURA

Protecting the confidentiality of a patient's health information used to be as simple as securing his chart from unauthorized eyes and holding discussions with or about him out of earshot of those who did not provide direct care.

Today, it is much more problematic. State laws and court rulings have created a number of exceptions to general confidentiality requirements. Public concern over sensitive issues such as HIV and genetic test results has led to a debate about special protections to ensure patients' privacy. And, technology has increased the ways patient information can be shared and, therefore, the number of people who have access to it. 3 Probs.

Every nurse, then, needs to know when and how to protect a patient's right to privacy—a right based on the U.S. Constitution and upheld by laws in all 50 states. Here's a look at the key issues and liability risks. Ans. 1

When are you compelled to disclose? Comp. Discl? 4

You have a legal duty to report certain situations in which the safety of the patient or the welfare of the public is considered at risk. Most jurisdictions require reporting of child and elder abuse and other illegal actions situations in which the patient may harm another, and communicable diseases. Because reporting requirements vary by state, you'll need to check with your risk manager or local statutes for specific provisions in your jurisdiction.

In general, however, as long as you report in good faith and according to the law, most statutes provide immunity from civil and criminal liability. And failure to report could subject you to a fine and disciplinary action. Ans. 2

Here are the four main exceptions to the rule of patient-provider confidentiality:

4 ex.   1. C + EA

Child and elder abuse. Every state requires nurses and physicians to report cases of suspected child abuse, neglect, and abandonment to the appropriate state agency or the police. A child is generally defined as anyone who is under the age of 18.

All states also require nurses in nursing homes to report cases of suspected elder abuse, neglect, and abandonment. Most states impose the same reporting requirement on nurses in other settings as well. The definition of an elderly patient varies—in Connecticut, for example, it's anyone who is over the age of 60—and some statutes don't specify an age.

Follow your employer's reporting policy. Document all observations of suspected abuse or neglect in the patient's chart, both physical (bruises, lesions, and so on) and psychological (fear or a withdrawn disposition).

ZOCA

Other criminal activity. All 50 states mandate that rape cases be reported to the police.[1] In some jurisdictions, narcotic use or evidence of violent crimes—such as gunshot or stab wounds—must be reported, as well.

Recently, Illinois and Oregon enacted laws that weaken the confidentiality rights of patients who are being treated for motor vehicle accident injuries. These states now allow health care providers to notify police about the results of blood or urine tests that show alcohol or drug levels above the legal limit. Maine has a similar law which states that if an RN or other provider knows or reasonably suspects that a patient who has been involved in a motor vehicle accident has been driving while under the influence of alcohol or drugs, she may report this to the police. So, nurses in these states who wish to report drivers who are drunk or high can do so without legal repercussions.

3. DP

Dangerous patients. If a patient tells you that he is going to harm another person, you may be obligated to disclose that information to protect the intended victim. That duty was established more than 20 years ago with the landmark Tarasoff case, in which the California Supreme Court found a psychotherapist liable for failing to warn a woman of his patient's plan to kill her—a plan that was carried out.[2]

If your patient makes such a threat, document it in his chart—in quotes and in his exact words, if possible—and question him further. If you believe the threat has merit, immediately inform your supervisor, risk manager, or the physician so that appropriate actions can be taken to avert harm.

4. CD

Communicable diseases. Certain infectious conditions must be reported to the appropriate state or local agency or health department. The most controversial disease on the reporting list: HIV/AIDS.

Every state requires the reporting of AIDS cases for epidemiological purposes—some require the reporting of the patient's name and address, while others prohibit the disclosure of any identifying data. Moreover, 28 states mandate the reporting—by name—of patients diagnosed with HIV. Some states also permit disclosure of a patient's HIV-positive status to third parties—say, a sexual partner or needle-sharing partner. However, many states allow only a physician or a public health officer—not the patient's nurse—to disclose this information. (See last month's Legally Speaking for more on HIV confidentiality parameters.)

When disclosure requires consent   Cons. Req.

Generally, informational data such as a patient's name, address, and dates of admission or discharge are not considered confidential information and therefore not protected by law. Information related to diagnosis, treatment, and prognosis, however, *is* considered confidential. Before disclosing this information to anyone other than members of the health care team—and unless otherwise mandated by law or a court order—you must obtain your patient's consent.

Verbal consent, either implicit or explicit, is usually sufficient to discuss your patient's health face-to-face with concerned family members or friends. You should try to avoid disclosing such information over the telephone, whenever possible. You never know who is really on the other end of the line.

But for anyone else—and especially when you're sending his actual medical records—obtain *written* authorization from the patient or, if he's unconscious, his representative.

In most cases, this can simply be a signed letter from the patient or a signed general consent form, such as the kind insurance companies use. In certain instances, however, a general letter or release is not enough.

Information related to a patient's HIV/AIDS status (other than that governed by the disclosure rules discussed earlier), psychiatric condition and drug or alcohol treatment receives special protection from disclosure under federal and state laws. You are prohibited from releasing any such information—including the patient's name or dates of admission or discharge—without your patient's *specific* consent.

As with a general release form, a patient's specific consent must be in writing, dated, and signed by him or his proxy. It must also state the purpose of the disclosure, the specific data to be revealed, to whom it can be revealed, who can make the disclosure, and how long the consent is valid.

When you're sending specially protected health information through the mail, make sure that it's accompanied by a statement of confidentiality, which prohibits the receiving party from revealing the information without the patient's consent. If you're disclosing the information verbally, you are not duty bound to recite this statement—but it certainly wouldn't hurt.

Currently, no special cloak of protection exists for another sensitive type of health information—genetic test results. But that is likely to change as more and more patients are tested for genes that mutate to cancer and other diseases.

Genetic information has raised fears by patients that their employers will discriminate against them and that insurance companies will deny or limit coverage. Some women who carry genes linked to breast or ovarian cancer are asking their doctors not to include this information in their medical records. Some doctors are complying with these requests, relying instead on their memories and pretending not to know any genetic information when they are dealing with insurers and other physicians.[3]

It's a thorny issue—what to do if a patient asks you not to chart potentially explosive information pertaining to diagnosis, prognosis, or treatment. At this point, it remains largely an ethical call that each health care professional must make for him- or herself.

Technology brings legal pitfalls, too   *Tech. Probs.*

Developments in communication technology have made the business of caring for patients more efficient. But using computers, fax machines, videotapes, and telephones to process, store, or transmit patient information has set the stage for security violations like never before.

Fortunately, the federal government has stepped in to help. The Health Insurance Portability and Accountability Act of 1996 mandates, among other things, that Congress establish privacy rules to manage electronic records within three and a half years of the law's enactment. These rules must stipulate that anyone with access to computerized health information be given training on maintaining confidentiality.

You should already be taking steps to ensure the privacy of electronic information. If you use a computer by the patient's bedside or at the nurses station, clear the screen after each use. Position the screen in a way that passersby cannot see it. And don't give your password to anyone.

Be sure to keep videotapes and backup computer disks—as well as paper records—in a secure place for the amount of time required by law. Never reuse tapes or disks because they may not be completely erased.

Avoid faxing medical information whenever possible. If it's unavoidable, verify the number you'll be sending the fax to and determine in advance that an authorized party will be on hand to receive it as soon as it comes in.

When providing health information over the phone, do so in a private area. Always verify to whom you are speaking and whether that person is entitled to information about a patient's health. If the party you are calling is not in, don't leave a message that reveals anything about a patient's condition. Instead ask to have the party you are calling return the call.

Of course, many breaches of confidentiality have nothing to do with technology at all. They occur when providers discuss confidential data in areas where they can be overheard. Hold all such discussions in a private location, away from unauthorized ears. When talking to a patient who is not in a private room, remember to keep your voice down.

Trust is a cornerstone of the patient-provider relationship. Making sure your patient's health information stays confidential will help you uphold that trust. <u>Understanding the exceptions to confidentiality rules in select situations will help put you on a course that's liability-free.</u>

References

1. Greve, P. A. (1990). Keep quiet or speak up? Issues in patient confidentiality. *RN, 53*(12), 53.

2. Tarasoff v. The Regents of the University of California, 13 Cal. 3d 177, 529 P.2d 553 (1974).

3. Kolata, G. (1997, February 4). Advent of testing for breast cancer genes leads to fears of disclosure and discrimination. *The New York Times*, p. C1.

Name _____

FINAL EXAM

1. In "Introduction to Physical Therapy," the major sections of the "Model Definition of Physical Therapy for State Practice Acts," are listed in which order?
   a. Consulting, researching, modifying, and functioning
   b. Examining, alleviating, preventing, and engaging in other activities
   c. Evaluating, functioning, debriding, and maintaining
   d. Promoting fitness, health, and quality of life

2. "The Birth of a New Profession" by Cullinan and Cullinan is written by
   a. retired radiologic technologists who know their subject first-hand.
   b. professional writers who have learned a great deal about radiology.
   c. co-directors of the American Society of Radiologic Technologists.
   d. people who are too young to have any idea about the history of radiology.

3. In her foreword to Leah Curtin's book, Margretta Madden Styles refers to the author as a
   a. nursing manager who knows how to crack the whip.
   b. dilettante who skims the surface of a vast pond.
   c. collector who never throws anything away.
   d. fine writer, pundit, and sage.

4. Which of the following is the best paraphrase of this marginal heading in Florence Nightingale's "Chattering Hopes and Advices": *Chattering hopes the bane of the sick?*
   a. Making light of the dangers of a person's illness is very destructive to the sick.
   b. Sick people may chatter when they are fearful or chilled.
   c. Chatting with the sick may help them to become more hopeful.
   d. Ruining the hopes for recovery of a patient is an unethical act.

5. According to Douglas in "Cultural Considerations for the African-American Population," the health efforts that will make the greatest strides in closing the disparity between health outcomes are
   a. never using first names in clinical settings, monitoring nonverbal communications, and not expecting eye contact.
   b. culturally sensitive, well developed, and well placed health education efforts.
   c. finding cures for AIDS, hypertension, and infant mortality.
   d. changing high-fat diets, lowering heart disease, and extending visitation privileges beyond immediate family.

6. In "Care of Patients with Pain," the author defines pain as
   a. a universal symptom, not specific to any one disease.
   b. whatever the person who is experiencing it says it is.
   c. a feeling of distress, suffering, or agony that is caused by stimulation of specialized nerve endings.
   d. all of the above.

7. According to the nursing definition of the term, what is an example of *empathy*?
   a. While she prepares to give an injection, the nurse tells the patient how sorry she is to have to cause any more pain.
   b. Feeling the patient's pain very strongly, a nurse refuses to administer any more intraspinal medication.
   c. Even though the patient seems to be improving steadily, the nurse consistently delivers the prescribed pain medication on time.
   d. Because the patient reacts stoically to pain, the nurse recognizes the patient's cultural background and suggests a milder form of medication.

8. In "Nurses' Judgments of Pain in Term and Preterm Newborns," the author's objective is to
   a. show nurses videotapes of newborns in pain.
   b. examine judgments of pain intensity and cues used by nurses in assessing pain.
   c. prove that the pain of preterm newborns is misassessed.
   d. review literature related to premature and full-term babies' pain.

9. In "Review of Literature on Culture and Pain of Adults, with Focus on Mexican-Americans," the authors see what implications for transcultural nursing practice?
   a. The extent to which a patient holds traditional beliefs should be the subject of further research.
   b. Nursing pain management should ask about the meaning a patient attaches to particular pain behaviors and the type of intervention desired by the patient.
   c. Pain assessment tools are not used frequently enough in current nursing practice.
   d. Quantitative research is needed to explore cultural beliefs.

10. In "Avoiding Opioid-Induced Respiratory Depression," the authors include which of the following risk factors for opioid-induced respiratory depression?
    a. Pulse, blood pressure, and adventitious sounds
    b. Age, renal dysfunction, and opioid tolerance
    c. History with opioids, concurrent medications, and opioid naiveté
    d. Dosages above 300 mg, postoperative medications, and ages under ten or over fifty

11. "The Golden Rule" provides a good example of
    a. teleological decision making.
    b. deontology.
    c. moral theories.
    d. intuitionism.

12. Which of the following is the best paraphrase of this sentence from "Ethical Perceptions of Parents and Nurses in NICU: The Case of Baby Michael": *Resolution of the dilemmas can be facilitated by the nurses' use of crisis intervention theory and caring processes?*
    a. Nurses can help resolve ethical problems by applying processes for caring and theories for crisis intervention.
    b. Solving nurses' dilemmas can be accomplished by using crisis intervention and caring techniques.
    c. Nurses who use crisis intervention and caring will facilitate dilemmas.
    d. Crisis intervention theory and caring processes can be used to resolve nurses' dilemmas.

13. In "Ethical Decision Making," four types of situations with varying relationships between ethics and the law are presented. Which of these are labeled "ambiguous"?
    a. Type 1: actions are both ethical and legal, and Type 2: actions may be considered ethical but not legal.
    b. Type 2: actions may be considered ethical but not legal, and Type 3: actions may be considered legal but not ethical.
    c. Type 3: actions may be considered legal but not ethical, and Type 4: actions are neither legal nor ethical.
    d. Type 1: actions are both ethical and legal, and Type 4: actions are neither legal nor ethical.

14. In "Caring for Pediatric Patients with HIV," Murphy and Famolare's purpose is to
    a. use direct quotes from nurses to illustrate ethical decision making.
    b. review literature on ethics as it relates to care of children with HIV.
    c. conduct formal research into nursing dilemmas.
    d. raise questions and show common dilemmas for the nurses surveyed.

15. In the article "When Language Is an Obstacle," the author uses which of the following to illustrate her point that some on-duty language restrictions are acceptable if they are motivated by a concern for patient safety?
    a. Title VII of the Civil Rights Act of 1965
    b. The EEOC's insistence that an individual's primary language is an essential characteristic of national origin
    c. A supervisor's ruling that employees must speak English at all times
    d. A California case in which concerns for patient safety were found to outweigh the Filipina nurse's civil rights

16. The authors of "Stress" identify three types of stress theories: stress as a response, stress as a stimulus, and a transactional or interactional view of stress. With which of these is Hans Selye identified?
    a. All of the theories
    b. The transactional or interactional view of stress
    c. Stress as a response
    d. Stress as a stimulus

17. In which stage of the General Adaptation Syndrome is the "flight-or-fight" mechanism initiated?
    a. The adaptation phase
    b. The end stage
    c. The alarm reaction
    d. The local adaptation syndrome

18. In assessing a client's stress, what three major areas should be considered?
    a. Demands, effects or human responses, and coping
    b. Stressors, the number of simultaneous demands, and the duration of the stressors
    c. Accident proneness, impaired speech, and crying
    d. Cognitive and behavioral coping strategies and defense mechanisms

19. Which of the following is the best summary of Lisa Robinson's article, "Stress and Anxiety"?
    a. Stress is difficult to define, but it includes psychobiologic variables, the influence of life events, and an interactional model. The psychophysiologic reactions are immediate. Thus, the focus should be on pharmacotherapy, psychotherapy, behavioral techniques, personality engineering, relaxation training, and biofeedback.
    b. Anxiety is the first sign of the stress response that may last several weeks and result in decreased resistance to disease. There are many strategies for preventing and moderating the stress response. The growth of nursing research on stress during the 1980s has provided four categories of coping with stress: cognitive, emotional, behavioral, and physical.
    c. Psychophysiologic signals are very important in stress research. The response has multiple foci. Three weeks after confrontation with the stressor neuroendocrine alterations occur. There are intervention and prevention studies that have influenced the nursing intervention strategies.
    d. Contemporary stress research focuses on psychobiologic phenomena in experience with a stimulus or situation that is appraised as aversive or unpleasant. Nursing research explores clinical interventions and preventive actions aimed at neutralizing adverse health effects secondary to stressful encounters.

20. In "Analyzing Job Demands and Coping Techniques," the authors' main purpose is to
    a. contrast two types of responses to stress.
    b. interview nurses under stress on a typical day.
    c. list successful coping skills for nurses to use.
    d. offer strategies for identifying and working with two groups of staff.

Reading and Remembering Test Four: Review

Observe the process you use in preparing to write a summary of the attached article [Mattera, M.D. (1997). Editor's memo. *RN,60*(7), 7].

1. Summarize the article, covering the main ideas and essential details in no more than five sentences.

2. Write an explanation of the process you used to study this article, revealing your knowledge of each phase of the reading process.

3. *BONUS:* Analyze the stress coping behaviors mentioned in the article according to the categories used by Lisa Robinson in her article "Stress and Anxiety."

EDITOR'S MEMO

Forgotten in the ER

DAVID BOONE, a past president of the Georgia Trial Lawyers Association, is an attorney in Atlanta. I thank him for sharing his story with our readers.

Here's a story you all need to hear:

I was lying on a gurney in a hallway of a very busy Florida hospital, wondering when someone would notice me. About two hours earlier, I'd been playing in a motel pool with my kids when I lost my balance, went under, and struck my head on the bottom. My neck flexed in an odd way. And now I had tingling sensations in my hands and arms.

The ER was crowded—Saturday night, a full moon. The first nurse I saw took a quick look at my bleeding head and told me to have a seat. She didn't ask how I'd been hurt. That seemed wrong, but it was busy. I did as I was told.

Some time later, another nurse took a look at me, heard how I'd hurt my neck and about the tingling sensations. She turned ashen and said she couldn't believe I didn't have a cervical collar on. She rummaged around but couldn't find one. So she had me lie on a gurney, wheeled me to the trauma room, and parked me outside.

People came and went. Some even asked one another, "Who's that guy?" Nobody stopped. I was afraid to move—I knew the risk of spinal injury.

So I lay there quietly, trying to relax and lower my blood pressure. I forced myself to breathe slowly and calmly. I knew I was relatively okay; I could still flex my fingers and toes. But I also knew that if I didn't receive treatment in the next few hours—with specific steroids—whatever damage my spinal cord had sustained could become permanent.

Finally someone spoke to me. It was a doctor. She looked puzzled. She wanted to know who I was and why I was there.

"My name is David Boone," I said. "I had a diving injury two hours ago. I have bilateral paresthesia. To me, it mimics a C-5, C-6 cervical injury, and I have yet to see a doctor."

"Are *you* a doctor?" she asked.

"No," I said, "I'm a medical malpractice attorney."

What happened next was like something out of a sitcom. Within minutes, though, I was being treated. And today, I'm just fine.

No, I didn't sue the hospital, and I'm not going to. They made a mistake and, once they discovered it, they corrected it. That's what professionals do.

But my story carries a reminder for every health care provider: Looks can be deceiving. Just because an accident victim is walking and talking doesn't mean he's okay. My only visible injury was a cut on the head. The first nurse I saw shouldn't have assumed that was all that was wrong.

I knew enough about spinal injury to keep myself calm and immobile until I got proper treatment. When the doctor finally arrived, I knew what to tell her. Few patients will be that knowledgeable. And what they don't know can hurt them—and you.

Answer Key for Final Exam

1.	b	11.	a
2.	a	12.	a
3.	d	13.	b
4.	a	14.	d
5.	b	15.	d
6.	d	16.	c
7.	c	17.	c
8.	b	18.	a
9.	b	19.	b
10.	c	20.	d

Scoring Guide for Reading and Remembering Process Test Four: Review

1. Summary
   - Mattera, the editor of *RN*, presents a letter from David Boone, an Atlanta medical malpractice attorney, as her editorial comment for July 1997.
   - Boone had been in the emergency room for two hours following a swimming pool accident in which he hit his head and twisted his neck.
   - Although he was experiencing some signs of neurological damage, he was receiving no treatment.
   - Remaining still and trying to stay calm, Boone was eventually discovered by a doctor to whom he explained his accident and symptoms in medical terminology.
   - Discovering that he was a malpractice attorney, the doctor put the emergency room staff into gear, treated his injury appropriately, and left Boone with no residual damage.

2. Explanation of the process, showing awareness of the phases:
   Phase 1: Before Reading
   - Previewing to discover that the article was an editorial column consisting of a letter with an introductory and concluding sentence. Also, estimation of difficulty as not very hard, and predictions about a nursing magazine's attitude/bias toward forgetting patients in the ER.
   - Developing a study plan for such a short piece isn't difficult, but reviewing the questions to be answered might have been a useful step.
   Phase 2: During Reading
   - Monitor comprehension, perhaps rereading to clarify who "I" is in the narrative.
   - Monitor reading efficiency by noting that the short article was fairly easy to read and may have been read at a faster than usual pace (although the testing conditions may slow some readers).
   Phase 3: After Reading
   - Because no long-term recall of the material is required, initial review may have been eliminated.
   - Some students may have used underlining or marginal note-making to prepare for the summary writing. Others may have begun drafting, returning to the editorial as needed to clarify concepts and to avoid overlap of wording.
   - Periodic recall is not appropriate or possible on this test item.

3. *BONUS*. Analysis of stress coping behaviors according to Lisa Robinson's article, "Stress and Anxiety," from the final section "Implications for Nursing Research and Practice."

Prevention through prediction and rehearsal, using reframing and redefinition: Boone probably had received some training in relaxation and other stress reduction techniques, but we don't have specific information on this. Mattera, the *RN* editor, may be attempting to help her readers rehearse more appropriate responses to patients by reading this story.

Behavioral coping strategies: Assertiveness and limit setting. Because of his need to remain still, Boone had few avenues of "behavior" available to him. He missed the first opportunity and didn't do very well with the second nurse, but he was ready by the time the doctor spoke to him on the gurney. He did avoid feeling like a victim, which is, perhaps, a form of limit setting.

Relaxation: Boone used this technique to stay calm and lower his blood pressure.

Physical coping strategies: Eating healthy foods and exercising. No evidence of these strategies.

Emotional coping strategies: humor. Boone was able to see the response of the medical team once he'd revealed his symptoms (and his profession) as like a "sitcom."

Cognitive coping strategies: cognitive restructuring. Although relatively unable to influence his surroundings, Boone avoided panic and increased his self-efficacy by developing a short, effective speech with which to capture the next caregiver's attention.

The hospital staff probably used every strategy in the book to avoid a malpractice suit!

A Word (or Two) on Vocabulary Development

Students planning a health career need to develop a strategy for managing vocabulary growth. They will encounter new technical terminology along with the usual spurt in general vocabulary growth experienced by college students. Thus, students need a method for using context to approximate meaning, for determining the best fit from all the dictionary definitions, for analyzing word parts, and for mastering the use of a new word in writing and speaking.

Asking students to note three new vocabulary words each week and to complete a vocabulary card for each is a practical way to guide students' vocabulary development. For these purposes, any word that occurs in a context (even a spoken sentence) is acceptable, but words taken from lists or the dictionary are not because they don't always come with a surrounding context. Context is critical to signal the relative importance of a word to the learner.

On one side of the card, students write down their word and signal its pronunciation. Asking students to copy down the dictionary's diacritical marks doesn't guarantee that they will know how to pronounce the word. Encourage them to find out how the word sounds and then make notes that will remind them of the pronunciation.

The other side of the card includes several items:

1. The sentence in which the word was encountered, including a brief bibliographical note, especially the page number of the book in which the word was found. If students make a mistake in copying the sentence, they may get a distorted idea of the meaning. With the page number noted, they can go back and confirm the sentence easily.

2. The meaning of the word. Although it might be useful to know the multiple meanings of a new word, the meaning as it is used in the original context is most important. There's a definite intellectual challenge in matching a dictionary's definition to its usage in a particular sentence.

3. The meaning of word parts and anything else interesting about the history of the word that will help in remembering it. Students will need considerable help in learning how to use the etymology provided in the dictionary.

4. A new sentence with enough context to make it clear that the word is used correctly. Students should try to use personal experiences and familiar names to aid in recall of the newly learned term.

Students turn in three new cards each week that the teacher quickly checks for accuracy and then returns. They also keep a list of the new words without any definitions. At the time of unit tests, each student gets his or her own vocabulary list from which to write a paragraph on a pre-announced topic. Family, sports, college, health careers, and pain are the kinds of topics that are familiar to students and yield an effective test of their mastery. The test is graded closely for accurate use and spelling, but a certain amount of leeway can be granted in the overall coherence of the passage; factual accuracy isn't a criterion at all! We once had a student write a totally convincing paragraph about her father's experiences on his national Olympic swimming team, but she was embarrassed to find that we thought it was true.

Learning about the meaning of word parts is also crucial for students in the health fields. Many lists of common Latin and Greek prefixes, roots, and suffixes are available. For developmental students who are not yet in a professional program, the lists of medically related word parts are very difficult. But learning the more common word parts also provides a powerful aid to vocabulary development. Learning useful word parts can also help students practice memorization. Memorization, though not fashionable, is a necessary skill for students in health careers. Flash cards can be used to drill, and involving family members in the practice may offer them an opportunity to be involved in a college education.

Some Ideas about Book Reports

Students in reading classes are often asked to make book reports. There's little doubt that the extra time spent reading helps students spend "time on task," which is requisite to improved performance. A list of titles is attached that might be useful in helping students find an interesting book to read. It's useful to have book reports reinforce the critical skills of summarizing and analyzing, and the form the report takes (a critical essay, a letter to a friend, or something else) is a matter of choice.

For students entering the health fields, the periodical report is also appropriate. For this project students choose one of the library's health-related periodicals for a report that will include an analysis of the format and features of the journal summaries of three course-related articles. Although each student reports on only one periodical, we often ask the class to form pairs or teams of classmates from whom they can seek advice and to whom they can offer support.

The project takes place over the course of a month. During the same time in class, students are being introduced to the concept of summary writing. An introduction to the features of periodicals and using general-interest magazines takes place in the classroom. A library trip to the periodical collection allows students to make a choice from the range of publications and to begin work. Over the next three weeks, students are encouraged to return to the library to check out additional issues of their journal in order to look for articles to copy and summarize. In the process, students look at multiple issues of the periodical and become familiar with recurring features, with the look and style of the publication, and with its difficulty/usefulness level. These observations culminate in a report in which the student describes the periodical and summarizes three articles that relate to some topic in *RSNAH:* health professions, pain, ethical/legal issues, stress. On the day reports are turned in, students are asked to share a brief comment about their periodical, offering at least a "thumbs up or down" about whether they would want to use the magazine for research in the future.

Part of the report is a statement about the assistance given to and by team members. Group study is a crucial survival skill for health majors, and this project gives developmental students a taste of collaborative effort.

One version of the report form is included.

Name _____

Description of Health Periodical

Title of Periodical:

Dates of the issues inspected:

How often is it published?   Where is it published?

Cost: Average length of an issue:

Pagination: Continuous in volume? _____   New in each issue? _____

Major sections/regular features:

Advertising included? If so, describe the kinds of advertisers:

Job vacancy notices included?   Yes _____   No _____

General Appearance:

Purpose/Intended Audience and Difficulty Level:

Summarize three articles that relate to a topic in *RSNAH:* professional issues, pain, ethical/legal issues, or stress. In your summary, include the main ideas and conclusions of the article plus a one-sentence personal reaction or evaluation. Don't write too much: All three summaries must fit on one page. Attach copies of the three articles.

Reading and Instructional Resources

The following are a few sources for reading about health-related issues. If you choose to assign outside reading, these may help your students find something of interest to them. A number of novelists with prior experience in medical occupations are currently publishing. Novels by Robin Cook, Michael Crichton, and P. D. James may have health-care settings and meet reading requirements for this assignment.

Books

Alcott, L. M. (1993). *Hospital sketches*. Cambridge, MA: Harvard University Press.
> The author, better known for her book *Little Women*, served as a nurse in Washington, D.C., during the Civil War. These sketches are based on her experiences. This book provides a view of nursing, influenced by Florence Nightingale, and an interesting comparison to the experiences of the English nurses in the Crimea.

Belkin, L. (1993). *First do no harm*. New York: Fawcett Crest.
> Based in Hermann Hospital in Houston, TX, the author describes the difficult daily decisions of doctors, patients, and their families.

Brown, M. (1992). *Nurses the human touch: The real-life experiences of registered nurses*. New York: Ivy Books.
> The author presents individual stories of nurses in different roles. Based on interviews, the chapters introduce the reader to a variety of career options for the registered nurse as they tell stories of nurses in those roles.

Carpinto, J. (1994). *On call*. Boston: St. Martin's Press.
> This book tells the story of three young doctors working in an inner-city hospital. There is routine and excitement as they work in the operating room, clinics, and the delivery room.

Close, W. T. (1995). *Ebola*. New York: Ivy Books.
> The author lived in Zaire for 16 years and worked to control the first outbreak of the virus in 1976. This book presents his personal experience with one of the most dangerous and deadly diseases currently known.

Cousins, N. (1979). *Anatomy of an illness as perceived by the patient: Reflections on healing and regeneration*. New York: W. B. Norton & Company, Inc.
> This is the story about the author's recovery from a serious collagen disease. A layperson who has led in the movement to improve health by using humor, he describes his own experience with the use of humor to aid in recovery.

de Kruif, P. H. (1954). *Microbe hunters.* San Diego: A Harvest/HBJ Book.
   de Kruif, a bacteriologist and pathologist, writes about medical mysteries and leaders in the discoveries in what is commonplace in medicine today. This is an interesting account of some of the important steps in medicine.

Heron, E. (1994). *Condition critical: The story of a nurse continues.* New York: Ivy Books.
   Describing her work as a critical care nurse, Echo Heron details events with humor and pathos. This book is a continuation of *Intensive Care.*

Heron, E. (1987). *Intensive care: The story of a nurse.* New York: Ivy Books.
   The author writes about how a nurse lives and works in the intense environment where patients are critically ill and every moment is a life-and-death struggle.

Lloyd, J. & Herman, E. B. (1995). *Dial 911.* New York: Ivy Books.
   Written by EMS/paramedics, this book provides both the male and female perspective of these roles.

M. & Moccia, P. (1993). *On nursing.* New York: National League for Nursing Press.
   An anthology of poems, biographies, essays, letters, articles, and stories about nursing.

McCarthy, C. (1995). *Learning how the heart beats: The making of a pediatrician.* New York: Viking Penguin.
   The author describes her experiences at Harvard Medical School and Boston's Children's Hospital. An interesting read for anyone interested in medicine with special interest for women hoping to become doctors.

Nuland, S. B. (1994). *How we die: Reflections on life's final chapter.* New York: Knopf.
   Winner of the National Book Award, this book addresses a subject of increasing interest to Americans as we become aware of the intensive efforts used to keep the dying alive. Because most deaths occur in hospitals, this surgeon-author wonders if death would be a less fearful process if it were brought out into the open. He proposes that if we view death as a biologic process that we allow to take its course, we would probably die more comfortably.

Nuland, S. B. (1992). *Medicine: the art of healing.* Hugh Lauter Leving Associates, distributed by Macmillan: New York, 1992.
   This art book includes essays that introduce the 48 works of art. Well written, this book provides a historical view of medicine from Hippocrates to more recent period.

Rouché, B. (1991). *The medical detectives.* New York: Truman Talley Books.
   Twenty-five detective stories of infectious outbreaks tell how the outbreaks were identified and treated. Each chapter is a separate story and allows reading as time is available. The language is clear as are the medical problems. This book is hard to put down.

Sacks, O. (1995). *An anthropologist on Mars: Seven paradoxical tales.* New York: Knopf.
   An account of seven persons with debilitating neurologic conditions whose conditions give insight into what makes one human. One of the tales is about an autistic woman with a Ph.D. Despite their handicaps, these persons have confronted life with courage and dignity.

Sacks, O. (1985). *The man who mistook his wife for a hat.* New York: Simon & Schuster.
   An account of a man who sought his help for a neurological disorder that caused him to lose contact with his world. Instead of recognizing individuals and items in his environment, he

was unable to make sense of the visual data despite enjoying music. An interesting book about a person with an unusual condition and the doctor who worked with him.

Sacks, O. (1989). *Seeing voices*. New York: Harper Perennial.
A book for those interested in the culture and history of the prelingually deaf. He describes the conflict between those who chose to use sign language and those who communicate verbally and use lip reading.

Sontag, S. (1978). *Illness as metaphor*. New York: Farrar, Straus & Giroux.
Sontag uses tuberculosis and cancer to compare and contrast metaphoric thinking about illness. The romantic view of the tubercular nineteenth-century patient is compared to the twentieth-century person with cancer who might have even brought it on himself/herself. It is an interesting comparison and best used as a point of discussion and analysis.

Verghese, Abraham. (1994). *My own country: A doctor's story of a town and its people in the age of AIDS*. New York: Simon & Schuster.
The autobiography is of a doctor of Indian descent, born in Ethiopia, who practices medicine in Johnson City, Tennessee. It describes the impact of AIDS on himself, his patients, their families, and the community. Well written; it is a book of sorrow but even more a book of hope.

Watson, J. (1968). *The double helix*. Philadelphia: Atheneum Publishers.
A classic, this short book describes the discovery of the structure of DNA. James Watson, 23 years old at the time of the discovery, writes about the scientific community involved in DNA research with humor and suspense.

Reference Books

Your library will probably contain some of these dictionaries and references. If not, you may want to place some of them on the order list. It will be important for your students to access a medical dictionary in order to deal with the medical terminology. If the health occupations programs in your institution require a particular reference, you may want to use that one as a primary reference.

Anderson, K. A. (Ed.) (1994). *Mosby's medical, nursing, & allied health dictionary*. St. Louis: Mosby-Year Book, Inc.

Cohen, B. J. (1994). *Medical terminology: An illustrated guide* (2nd ed.). Philadelphia: Lippincott.

Collins, C. E. (1996). *Modern medical language*. St. Paul, MN: West Publishing Co.

Firkin, B. G. (1996). *Dictionary of medical eponyms* (2nd ed.). Philadelphia: Parthenon Publishing.

Goldfarb, B. (1997). *Health care defined: A glossary of current terms*. Baltimore: Williams & Wilkins Co.

Kiley, R. (1996). *Medical information on the Internet: A guide for health professionals*. New York: Churchill Livingstone.

O'Toole, M. T. (Ed.) (1997). *Miller-Keane encyclopedia & dictionary of medicine, nursing & allied health* (6th ed.). Philadelphia: W. B. Saunders.

Pickett, J. & Pritchard, D. F. (Eds.) (1995). *The American heritage Stedman's medical dictionary.* Boston: Houghton Mifflin Company.

Spiegl, F. (1996). *Fritz Spiegl's sick notes: An alphabetical browsing book of medical derivations, abbreviations, mnemonics and slang for the amusement and edification of medics, nurses, patients, and hypochondriacs.* Pearl River, N.Y.: Parthenon Publishing.

Stedman, T. L. (1990). *Stedman's medical dictionary* (26th ed.). Baltimore: Williams & Wilkins.

Stedman. T. L. (1996). *Stedman's medical speller* (2nd ed.). Baltimore: Williams & Wilkins.

Thomas, C. L. (Ed.) (1997). *Taber's cyclopedic medical dictionary* (18th ed.). Philadelphia: F. A. Davis.

Journals

If you choose to have students do a periodical report, this list may be a useful starting point for a list of your library's holdings. Even if you do not use the report format, you may want to arrange a library tour to let students see some of these health-related publications.

AANA Journal (American Association of Nurse Anesthetists)
American Journal of Medical Technology
American Journal of Medicine
American Journal of Nursing
American Journal of Respiratory and Critical Care Medicine (formerly, *American Review of Respiratory Disease*)
Anesthesiology
AORN Journal (Association of Operation Room Nurses)
Applied Radiology
Cancer Nursing
Choices in Respiratory Management (formerly, *Respiratory Management*)
Clinical Laboratory Science
Critical Care Medicine
Diagnostic Imaging
Emergency Medicine
Harvard Health Letter
Heart and Lung
Hospital Medicine
International Nursing Review
JAAMT: Journal of the American Association for Medical Transcription
JAMA: Journal of the American Medical Association
JCU: Journal of Clinical Ultrasound
JOGNN: Journal of Obstetric, Gynecologic and Neonatal Nursing
Journal of Allied Health
Journal of Diagnostic Medical Sonography
Journal of Gerontological Nursing
Journal of Nursing Administration
Journal of Nursing Education

Journal of Practical Nursing
Journal of Psychiatric Nursing
Journal of Psychosocial Nursing
Journal of the American Dietetic Association
Journal of Transcultural Nursing
Journal of Ultrasound in Medicine
Journal of Vascular Technology
MCN: American Journal of Maternal Child Nursing
Medical Laboratory Observer
Medical Ultrasound
Modern Hospital
New England Journal of Medicine
Nursing
Nursing and Health Care
Nursing Clinics of North America
Nursing Forum
Nursing Life
Nursing Management
Nursing Mirror (merged with *Nursing Times*)
Nursing Outlook
Nursing Research
Nursing Times
Nursing Update
Patient Care
Pediatric Nursing
Physical Therapy
Professional Medical Assistant
P T Bulletin
Radiography Today
Radiologic Technology (title changed to *X-Ray Technician*, V. 32–34, May 1963. Title changed
    back to *Radiologic Technology* V. 36, July 1964.)
Regan Report on Nursing Law
Respiratory Care
Respiratory Management (formerly, *Respiratory Therapy*)
RN
Supervisor Nurse
Surgical Rounds
Surgical Technologist
Today's Surgical Nurse (formerly, *Today's OR Nurse*)

Multimedia

Multimedia resources are being introduced to the market almost daily. If your institution or health occupations programs have a multimedia lab(s), you may have these references available. They may become invaluable to you as well as to your students.

Dorland's electronic medical speller (Single User Diskette). (1996). Philadelphia: W. B. Saunders Company.

Ethical dilemmas and legal issues in care of the elderly (Level III Interactive Videodisc). New York: American Journal of Nursing Co., Educational Services Division.

Medical spellchecker (Diskette). (1996). New York: Obelisk Interactive.

Medical terminology: The language of health care (CD-ROM). Baltimore: Williams & Wilkins Co.

Mosby's medical encyclopedia (CD-ROM). (1995). Cambridge, MA: Softkey.

Rndex student edition (Computer Software). (1997). Albany, NY: DelMar.

Stedman's electronic medical dictionary 3.0 (Diskette and CD-ROM). Baltimore: Williams & Wilkins Co.

Internet Resources

The newest source of health occupation resources can be found on the Internet. A problem that you and your students need to be aware of is that the sites move or disappear without warning. There are so many good sites; your students, no doubt, will provide you with any number of good addresses.

Students also need to use judgment about what they read. Not everything on the Net is accurate information, and this is often a difficult concept for the novice to accept.

General Health Care Resources

American Pain Society	http://www.ampainsoc.org
American Physical Therapy Association	http://www.apta.org
Careers in Health Care	http://www.cbbn.com/sierra.htm
Centers for Disease Control and Prevention	http://www.cdc.gov
Dee's Pain Management Page	http://www.web-shack.com/dee
Online Clinical Calculator	http://www.intmed.mcw.edu/clincalc.html
Virtual Hospital	http://vh.radiology.uiowa.edu
World Health Organization	http://www.who.org

Nursing Sites

InterNurse	http://www.wp.com/InterNurse
Critical Care Nurse Snapshots	http://134.192.4.195/students/~jkohl/scenario/opening.htm
MedWeb: Nursing	http://www.gen.emory.edu/MEDWEB/keyword/Nursing.html
Nursing and Health Care Resources	http://www.bath.ac.uk/~exxrw/nurse.html

Nursing Center	http://www.nursingcenter.com
Nursing Index	http://www.lib.umich.edu/tml/nursing.html
Perioperative	http://www.aorn.org/nsgtoday/internet/links.htm
The Virtual Nursing Center	http://www-sci.liv.uci.edu/HSGNursing.html
Too Live Links	http://www.vgernet.net/toolive/links.html

Transparency Masters for *Reading Strategies for Nursing and Allied Health*

Reading and Remembering: A 3-Phase Process

Phase 1: *Before Reading*

GOAL 1: Get oriented to the text, the author, the assignment, and the scope and organization of the information

TECHNIQUES

1. Preview new materials and assignment
2. Estimate the difficulty of the material, and improve your background knowledge
3. Ask questions or make predictions about the information
4. Look up significant terms that are not defined in the text
5. Check for bias in the author or reader

GOAL 2: Develop a study plan

TECHNIQUES

1. Decide which parts of the text relate to objectives
2. Divide the assignment into smaller parts
3. Decide when to work on each part

Phase 2: *During Reading*

GOAL 3: Monitor comprehension and achievement of purpose

TECHNIQUES

1. Use understanding of main ideas, details, and paragraph organization
2. Stop at the end of sections to check achievement of outcome goals and to underline main ideas
3. Use alternate strategies or return to appropriate technique in Phase 1

GOAL 4: Monitor reading efficiency

TECHNIQUES

1. Adjust rate to purpose and difficulty
2. Evaluate study efficiency

Phase 3: *After Reading*

GOAL 5: Check initial recall of relevant information

TECHNIQUES

1. Review the whole assignment by self-testing or answering review questions
2. Return to appropriate technique in Phase 1 or 2 to restudy

GOAL 6: Organize relevant information for recall

TECHNIQUES

1. Make notes, outline, summarize, jot down questions
2. Look up and learn new terminology discovered during reading
3. Think critically about what you have learned
4. Apply principles to situations

GOAL 7: Test recall of relevant information periodically

TECHNIQUES

1. Review notes without rereading text
2. Predict and answer possible test questions

A Process for Reading and Remembering

Phase 1: *Before Reading*

GOAL 1:

Get oriented to the text, the author, the assignment, and the scope and organization of the information

TECHNIQUES

1. Preview new materials and assignment
2. Estimate the difficulty of the material, and improve your background knowledge
3. Ask questions or make predictions about the information
4. Look up significant terms that are not defined in the text
5. Check for bias in the author or reader

GOAL 2:

Develop a study plan

TECHNIQUES

1. Decide which parts of the text relate to objectives
2. Divide the assignment into smaller parts
3. Decide when to work on each part

A Process for Reading and Remembering

Phase 2: *During Reading*

GOAL 3:

Monitor comprehension and achievement of purpose

TECHNIQUES

1. Look for main ideas, significant details, and paragraph organization
2. Stop periodically to check achievement of outcome goals and to underline main ideas
3. Use alternative strategies or return to an appropriate *before-reading* technique in Phase 1

GOAL 4:

Monitor reading efficiency

TECHNIQUES

1. Adjust reading rate to purpose for reading and to difficulty of the text
2. Evaluate the efficiency of your study strategies

A Process for Reading and Remembering

Phase 3: *After Reading*

GOAL 5:
Check initial recall of relevant information

TECHNIQUES
1. Review the whole assignment by self-testing or answering review questions
2. To restudy, return to an appropriate *before-reading* or *during-reading* technique

GOAL 6:
Organize relevant information for review

TECHNIQUES
1. Underline, make notes, outline, summarize, and/or jot down questions
2. Look up and learn new terms discovered during reading
3. Think critically about what you have learned
4. Apply principles to real-life situations

GOAL 7:
Periodically test recall of relevant information

TECHNIQUES
1. Review notes without rereading the text
2. Predict and answer possible test questions

Three Types of Information to Look for in Previewing a New Textbook

1. Information Explaining the Book to the Reader

To find this information, look at the following:

- title page (one of the first pages of the text, containing the title, author, and publisher. The back of this page contains useful data on the date of publication)
- introduction (a lengthy guide to the book written by the author)
- foreword (a short introduction usually written by an expert in the field, other than the author)
- preface (an author's informal statement about the organization of the text, often including acknowledgments)
- acknowledgments (the author's expression of appreciation for those who helped in the preparation of the book)

2. Information about the Author

Look for these features:

- a short biography of the author, highlighting qualifications for writing the text, usually located in the front of textbooks
- dedication (an offering of the book to someone whom the author loves or respects), located at the front of the book

3. Organizational and Supplementary Information

Take a look at these features:

- table of contents (a more or less complete listing of chapters and topical headings, located in the front of the book)
- index (an alphabetical list of topics in the text along with the page numbers on which they are discussed, located at the end of the book)
- glossary (specialized definitions of terms used in the text, located at the end of a chapter or at the end of the text before the index)
- appendix (supplementary material at the end of the text including conversion charts, lists, and other useful information)

Calculating Elapsed Time

	Stop time:	8:10 PM
minus	Start time:	7:00 PM
	Total time:	1:10 minutes

	Stop time:	9:00 PM
minus	Start time:	7:15 PM
	Total time:	1:45 (remember that 9:00 is the same as 8:60; don't try to borrow 100 minutes!)

Previewing an Article

- article title and series heading, if available

- author identification

- introductory paragraph(s)

- headings

- photographs with their captions, other graphic aids

- concluding paragraph(s)

Organizational Patterns

comparison/contrast: showing similarities and differences

cause/effect: showing causes and/or results

process/time order: showing the sequence of steps in an action or in a series of events

listing: showing examples of a principle or concept with the order of presentation being more or less arbitrary—or at least not organized by one of the other patterns

"Care of Patients with Pain" Objectives

1. Define pain.

2. Describe physiologic and psychological reactions to pain stimuli.

3. Compare and contrast three different types of pain.

4. Describe common biases and myths about pain.

5. Assess pain in assigned patients, fully appreciating the subjective nature of pain.

6. List at least seven nursing interventions other than the administration of analgesics for the relief of pain.

7. Select nursing interventions appropriate for each type of pain experience.

8. Evaluate the effectiveness of measures used for the management of pain in assigned patients.

Editor's Outline Format	Author's Headings and Subheadings
Objective	Purpose of the Research
	Literature Review
Design	Methods
	Population and Setting
Setting	Instrumentation
	The instrument
	Establishing validity and consistency
Participants	Procedure
Interventions	Results
	Hypothesis 1
	Hypothesis 2
Main Outcome Measures	Discussion and Nursing Implications
Results	Limitations
	Recommendations for Further Research
Conclusions	Conclusions
	Acknowledgment

Three Reading Strategies

Skimming: rapid coverage of the whole article to confirm the ideas from the summary outline, focusing on "high yield" locations such as first sentences, last sentences, introduction, and conclusion

Selective Reading: thorough reading of only limited parts of the article, omitting those which are unlikely to yield information related to purpose

Comprehensive Reading: careful reading of the entire text when thorough understanding and recall are the goals